TALIA NEPPER

Unveiling Motherhood: Poems of Postpartum Resilience

This book was professionally typeset on Reedsy.
Find out more at reedsy.com

Contents

V   Love, Marriage, A Baby in a Carriage...Then What?

Introduction

I spent my whole life dreaming of being a mom. And then suddenly it was happening to me, and NONE of it was how I expected. And I kept asking, "Why does nobody talk about this? Why did nobody tell me?"

This book of poems is my way of sharing my story in an effort to help other moms who might be experiencing similar thoughts. You are not alone.

* * *

Before you begin reading, I'd like to offer a trigger warning that this book contains content involving difficult pregnancies, traumatic births, near death experiences, c-sections, postpartum mental illness, abuse, and divorce. Some swear words are present throughout the writing.

* * *

To give a little back story, I will share with you the important details of my journey.

When I became pregnant with my son, I was truly shocked as I thought I could never have children due to some of my own health issues. I was immediately elated. But that quickly waned when I found out I was in a high risk pregnancy, with hyperemesis gravidarum, and I was more sick than I had ever been in my life.

I was also terrified from the beginning that either the baby or I wouldn't survive the pregnancy or birth. I wish I could say I was just overthinking it, but when I found out I was pregnant, I had a doctor tell me that it would be a miracle if we both survived. And that stuck with me in the most awful way. I don't think I enjoyed a single minute of my pregnancy because I was so filled with fear.

After a horrendous pregnancy, I endured a life altering birth. I had hoped desperately for a natural birth and went all the way to 42 weeks pregnant. In the very last moment before I was about to go to the hospital to be induced, labor began in a hurried, anguishing frenzy. For the next 24 hours, I would experience relentless contractions less than a minute apart, at an awful and unbearable intensity. About 14 hours in, I begged to be transferred to the hospital from the birth center as I was in too much agony. After receiving an epidural, I found out I was suffering from an infection, Chorioamnionitis.

My body went into survival mode, and my son went into distress. By morning, I became unresponsive and unable to speak or move. I could only mumble, and the only words I could get out were, "I need you to take him out or I am going to die."

I was not believed. I was ignored. And by the time they finally took action, I was hanging on death's doorstep with a very serious septic infection. I was taken for an emergency c-section, of which I only remember terrifying snippets. I did not witness my son's birth. I saw him only through flickering lids, and I don't remember meeting him, much less the rest of his first week of life.

And the shame I carried from that was immense. I felt I had failed him. I felt I failed myself. I blamed my body for the significant betrayal. As a result, I struggled deeply to connect with my son.

My physical recovery felt insurmountable.

I somehow felt like a stranger in my own body.

Though there was only a tiny baby between us, there suddenly was an entire world between me and my husband.

I watched myself disappear. I crumbled into darkness.

Though people will tell you the postpartum period only lasts for the first three months of the baby's life, unfortunately for many, postpartum anxiety and depression and rage, among other postpartum mental health illnesses, do not follow the same timeline. This was the reality for me.

For the first nine months, I was in a very deep hole, and when I found out I was unexpectedly and fearfully pregnant at nine months postpartum, I hit rock bottom again.

I barely made it through another pregnancy, both mentally and physically, and suffered through much of it alone. Some of this was in part due to my pregnancy being in the heart of the pandemic, 2020-2021. And unfortunately, the other part was because I was becoming more and more isolated in my marriage.

Though I won't go into details, I had another very traumatic birth, another year of postpartum depression, with an extra spicy side of anxiety and OCD.

I floundered a lot.

I thought it would never end. But it did. Eventually, it did.

With the help of an art therapist, a trauma therapist, an amazing psychiatrist, and some other resources which I relied on heavily, I finally found the light.

* * *

During that postpartum time period, I turned to the only ways I could manage to sort through my grief and trauma: art, writing, and therapy. This book is a result of that journey.

I have since been on a mission to live my life out loud. I suffered in silence for far too long, and it almost ended me.

These are my very raw, unfiltered, honest, and sometimes ugly thoughts. I give fair warning that this book is not filled with the joyful moments that so many parents often share. Most of these feelings were awful, and a lot of my journey was not happy. But I am finding my way again into the person who I want to be, and while it is not perfect and moments are difficult, I'm finding contentment and purpose again.

It is my true hope that through these poems, I can help other moms see that they are not alone, they are not crazy, and they are not mad. They are dealing with something very real.

Yes, motherhood can be incredibly amazing, rewarding, and so gratifying you feel your heart will burst. But it's also okay to acknowledge that being a parent is hard. Really hard...especially at the very beginning.

Please know that good moms aren't the ones who don't struggle. They're simply the ones who do the best they can, for their babies AND for themselves.

* * *

P.S. While it is not the main focus of the book, art therapy became a life saving discovery in the midst of my healing. The photos included depict my original works that have been created along my journey on the way to recovery. They are separate from the poems and do not correlate directly in most cases.

I

Pregnancy

Belly Brushes

My hands keep finding my belly,
Fingers brushing against my skin,
Wondering if you're actually there.
But you don't feel real.
None of it does.
I know you're a miracle.
I want to believe in you.
But what if I never meet you?
The thought is too much to bear.

* * *

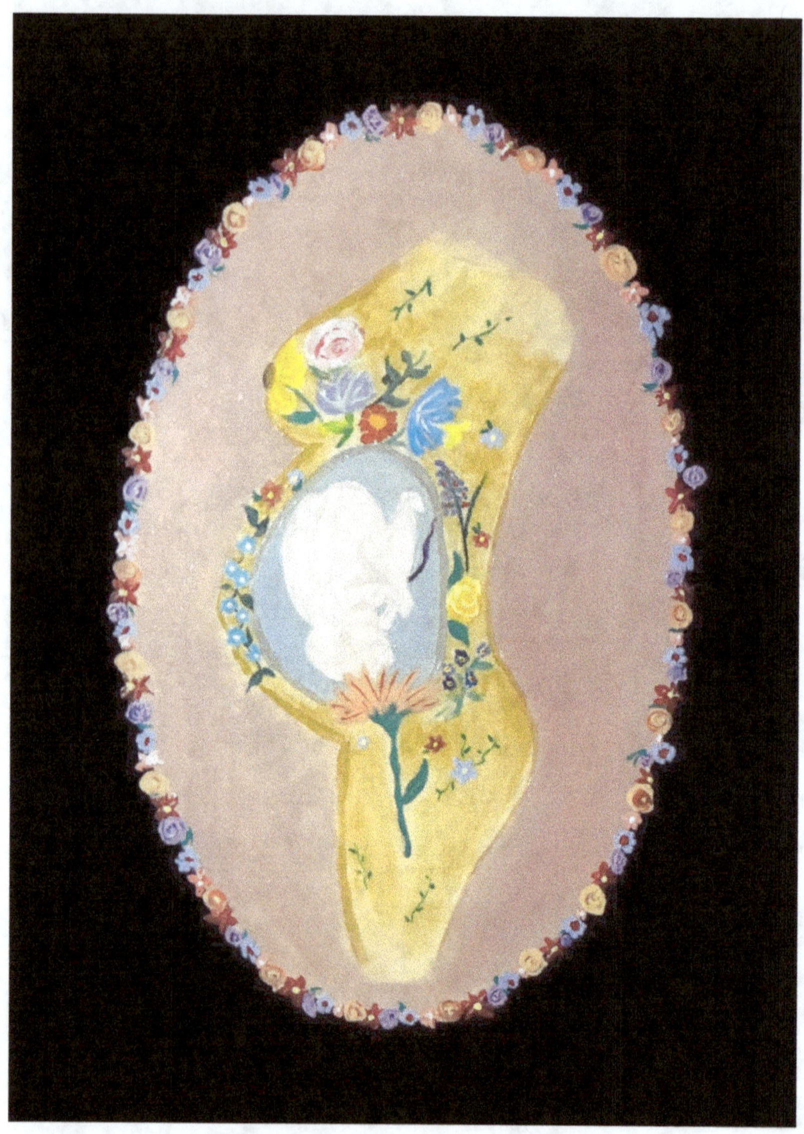

"Blooming", Acrylic, 9" x 12", 2020

Sick for a cause

I puke again.
That's how I know you're there.
But otherwise, I have no proof,
I just gasp for air.

I retch, heave, and cry like a kid,
You're the size of a grain rice,
But nausea and sickness persist,
"Oh god, don't mention the spice."

I gag, and wonder
how I'm supposed to glow
But somehow instead
green chunks I blow.

I curl in bed, unable to move,
If I do, my insides will revolt again.
If you're in there,
Can't we be friends?

I promise to grow you well,
If you'd just let me eat.

I snack out of necessity,
But you have me beat.

Morning sickness,
Afternoon and night,
Really every second of the day,
Is such a fight.

You're worth it,
A million times over, I know,
But I never knew
A baby was this hard to grow.

* * *

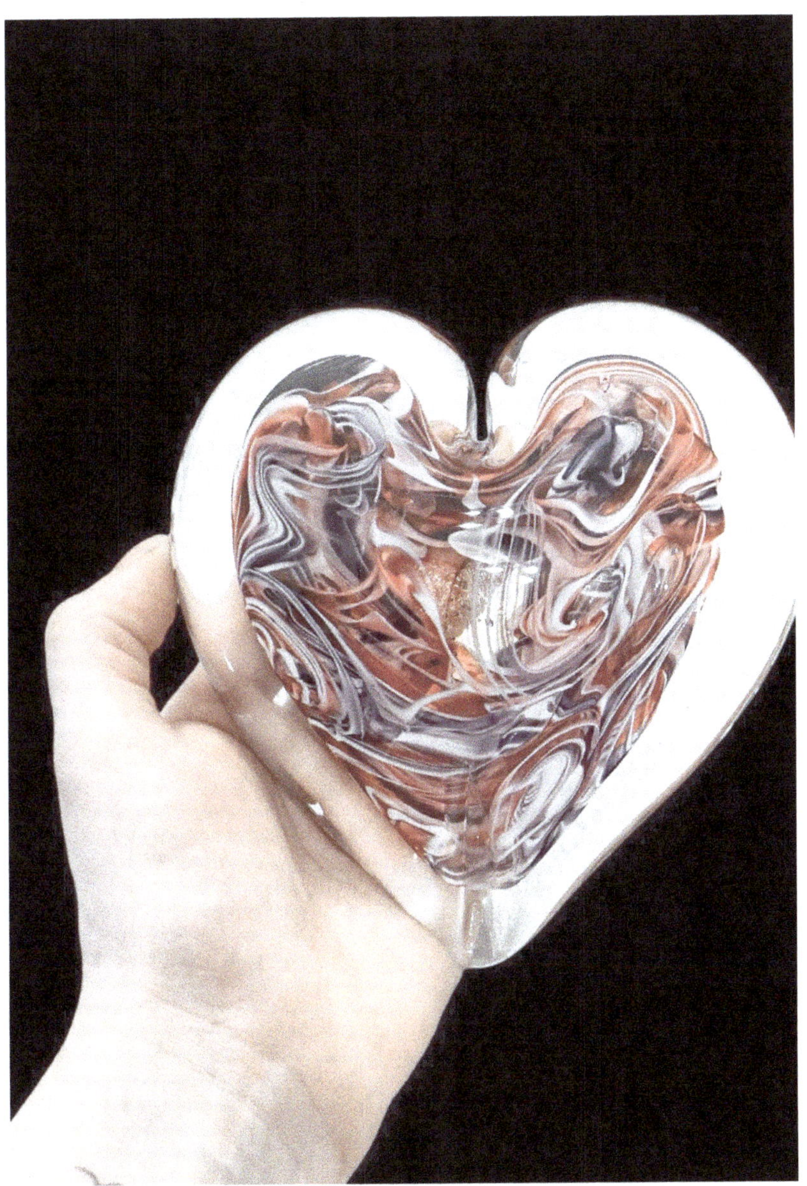

"They replaced my heart", blown glass, 2023

Beating for you

I heard your heartbeat today,
and I swear, for the first time in my life,
I felt mine beating with a purpose, too.

* * *

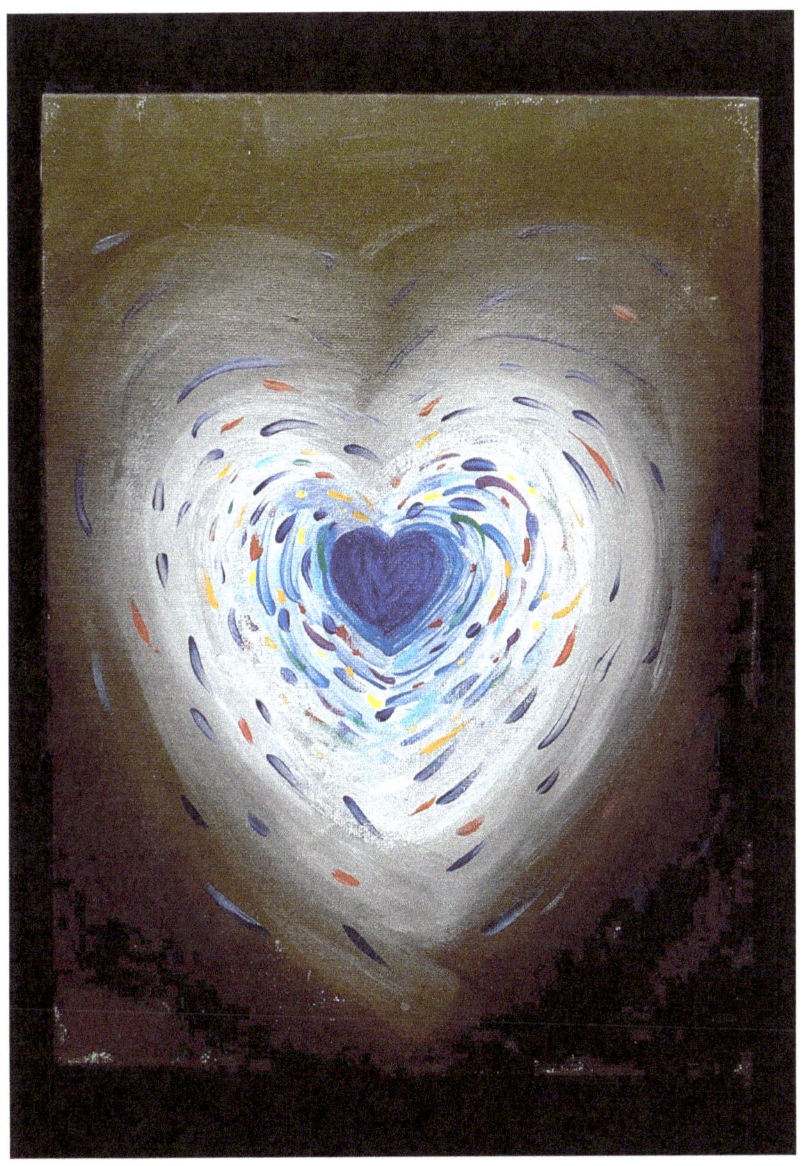

"The further apart, the darker my heart", Acrylic, 9" x 12", 2020

Hiccups Heaven

My belly jumps in a rhythmic beat,
Gosh, your hiccups are so sweet.
They make me laugh and giggle, too.
I get a glimpse of the little you.

Your kicks dance around,
And with my hands they are found.
I watch with awe and disbelief,
Those really are your tiny feet.

* * *

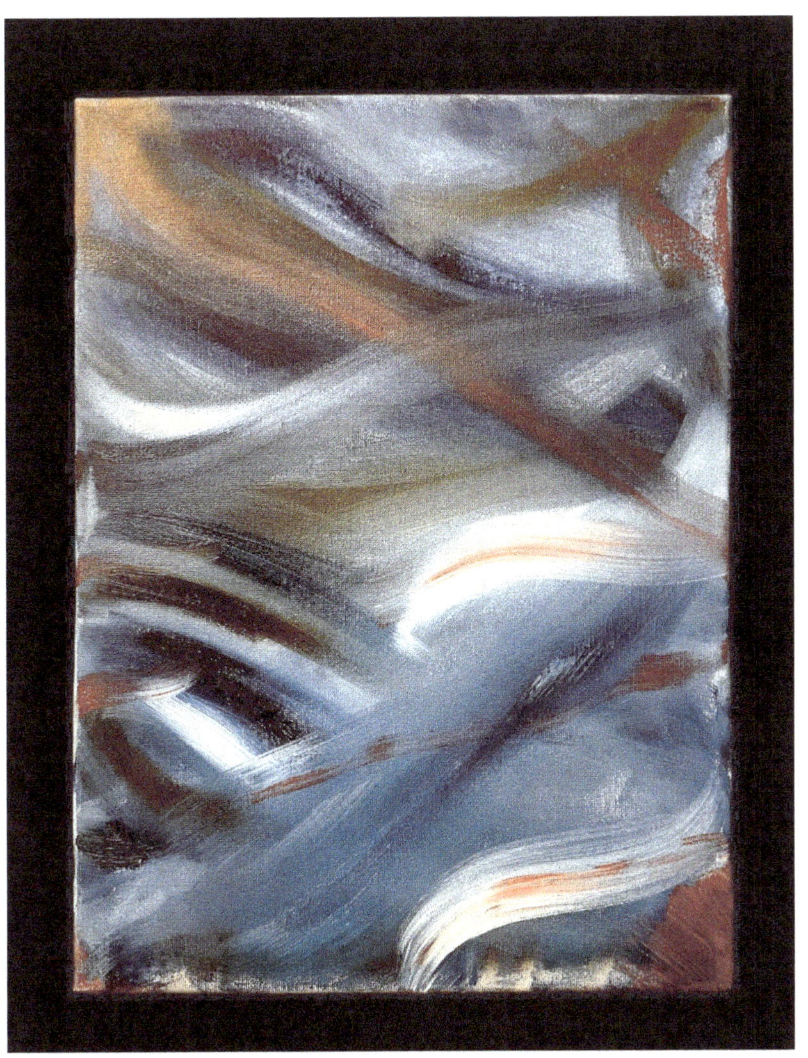

*"**Water Blur**", Oils, 12" x 16", 2019*

Foreshadowing

I dreamed my whole life about being a mom,
Only to find out I might never know the depths
Of a love so great.

And to find you were coming,
I was ecstatic yet terrified,
Because I was told we might not make it,
Maybe not you, maybe not me.

So I faced each day with fear in my heart,
That I would lose you,
Before I even got to meet you,
That I would lose me, too.

"I'm going to die," I told myself.
And maybe it was a knowing,
Maybe it was foreshadowing,
Perhaps I created it into existence,
But I never could have imagined how close I'd come.

* * *

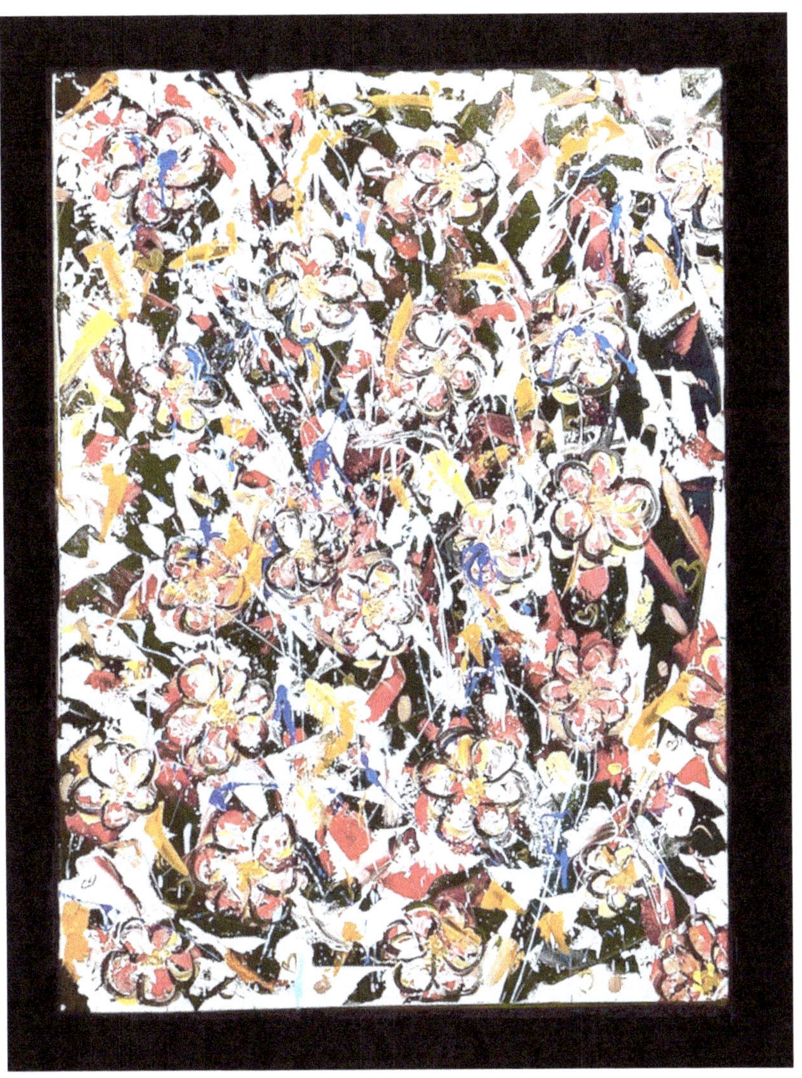

"Forget Me Not", Acrylic, 36" x 48", 2023

Scrawled Stripes

I watch the etched lines form up my belly,
And I somehow feel disappointed.
My body is changing so rapidly,
And though I know it's a miracle,
I can't keep up my facade.
Because this body doesn't feel like mine.
It feels like yours.

And while I want to be selfless
and say I don't care about the stupid stripes,
I find myself gasping at their deep purple color,
And the way the creep around the skin,
That was once smooth.
The skin that was once mine.

But that skin isn't mine anymore.
It's yours.
And I surrender.
Because who cares about about tiger stripes,
When I get to hold you at the end of this?

* * *

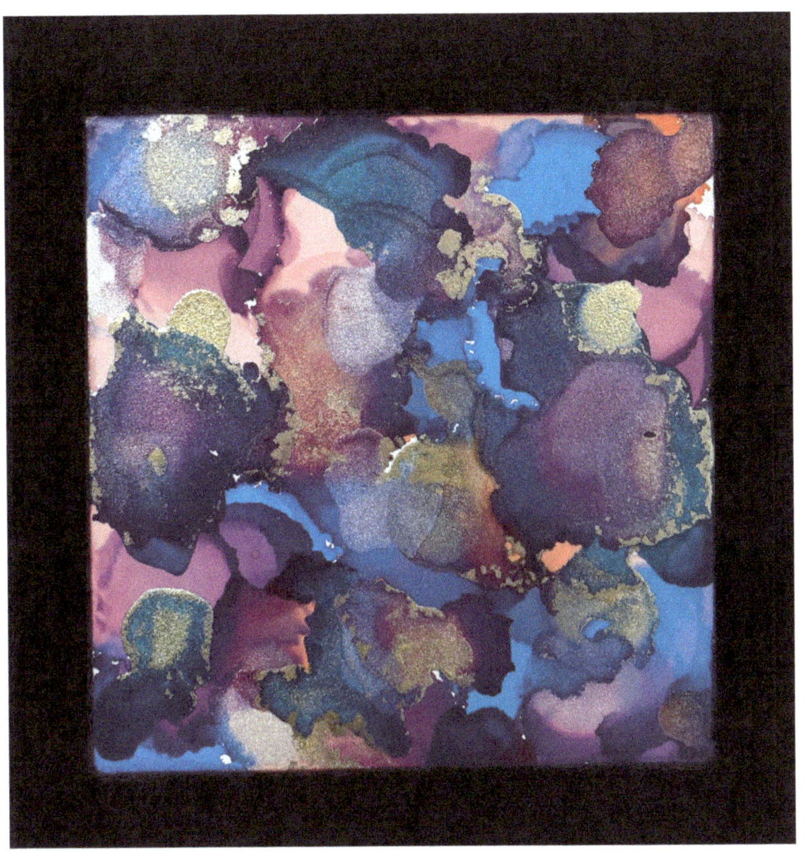

*"**Gemstones**", Alcohol Inks, 4" x 4", 2021*

An ode to my back

Oh sweet back, you once were strong,
But the weight of this baby has dragged you along.
I feel your restless, aching pull,
And in my hips, it feels so full.
I walk just around the block,
In this oversize maternity smock.
You ache and groan, and it hurts so bad,
But other people don't always get this,
"So just be glad."

***

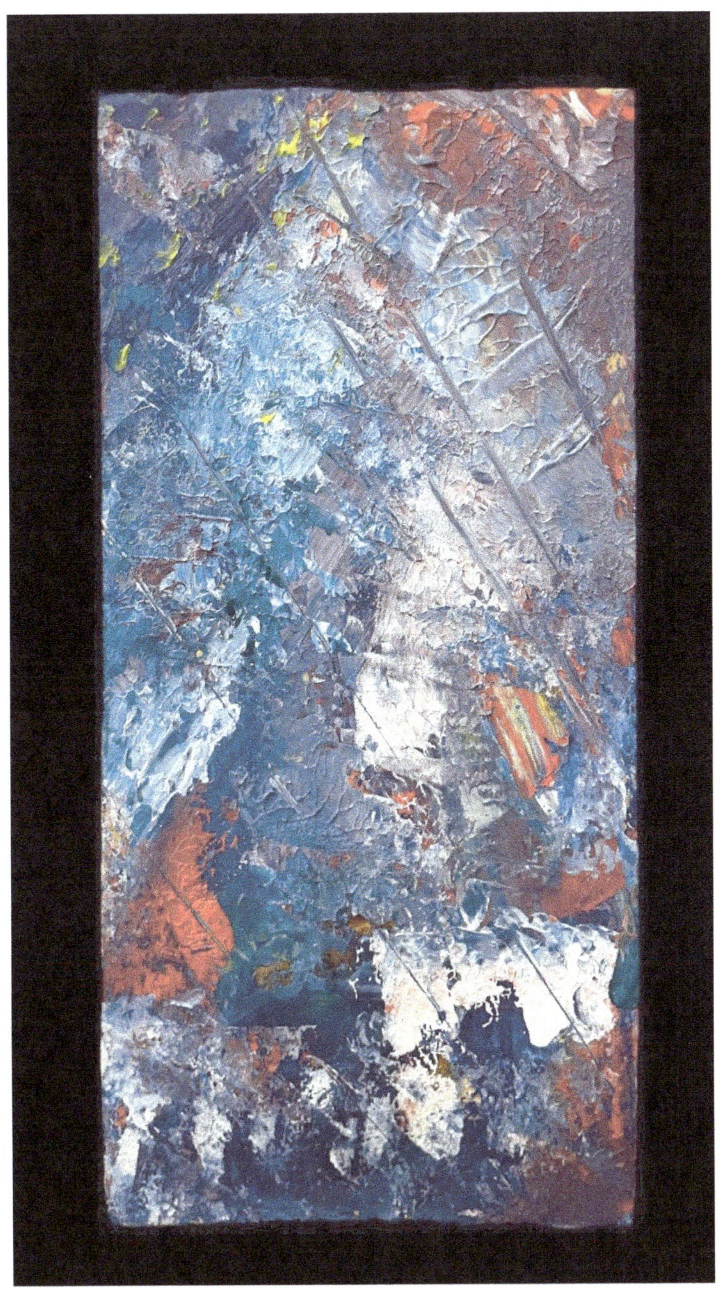

"Can anyone hear me?", Acrylic, 4" x 7", 2019

Ignorance is not bliss

"Is it twins?" they laugh and scoff,
And I just want to tell them to bugger off.
"No, just one," I sweetly say,
Underneath my heavy sway,
But they ask again, "Are you sure there's not two?
You look like you should be due!"
And I know it's only ignorant quips,
But I can't help but purse my lips.
"Yes, just one, I'm three months away,
Have a lovely fucking day."

* * *

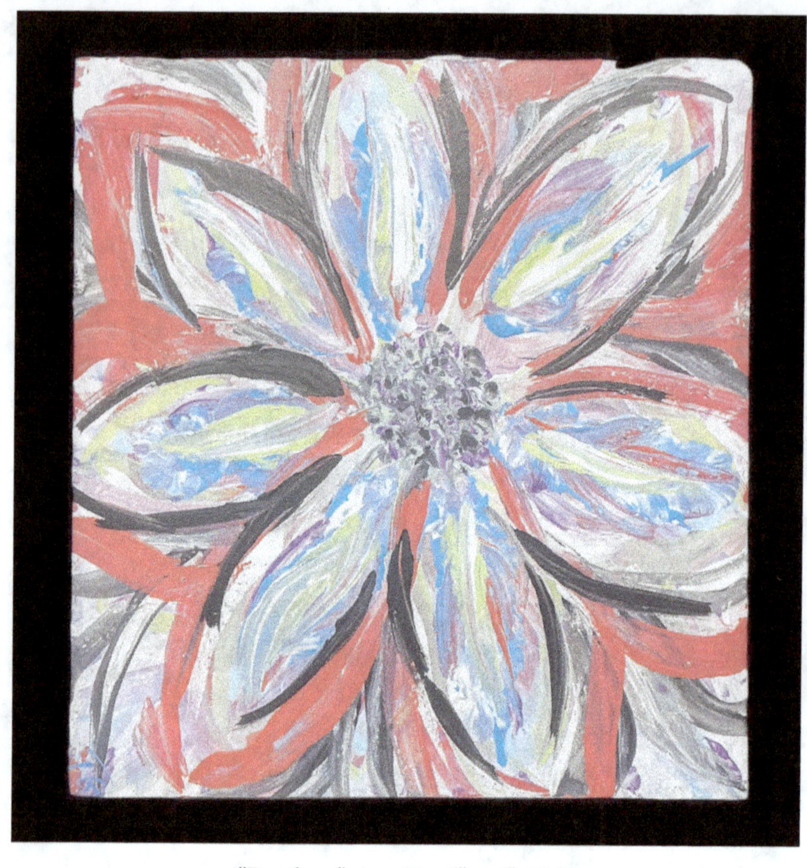

*"**Daphne**", Acrylic, 6" x 6", 2023*

Moms don't get to complain

"Don't complain, you have it so good,
You're not enjoying it how you should."

But I'm exhausted and in agony and nauseous for days,
Isn't that okay to say?

"No, no, be thankful for what you've got,
Don't complain, not everyone has this shot."

I know that, I do. I swear I'm grateful.
But why do you have to be so hateful?

"You don't know how good you have it,
Your negativity I won't permit."

I am blessed, that's true, I've always wanted this.
But please, just let me say it out loud.
This pregnancy has thrown me into the abyss.

* * *

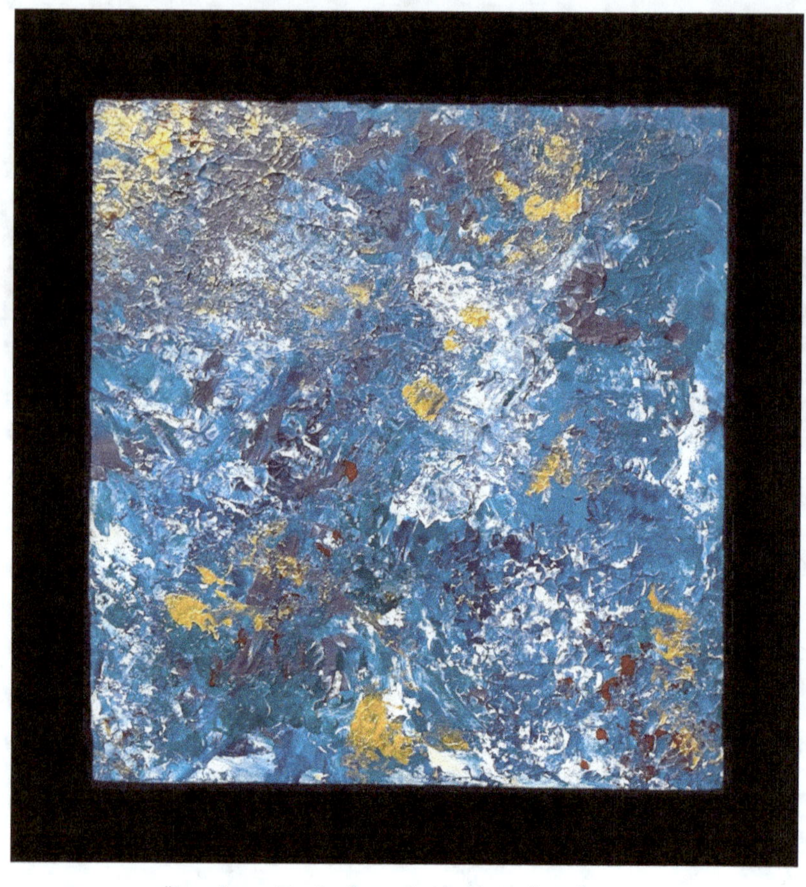

"Precious Turbulence", Acrylic, 7" x 7", 2020

Halted

Your feet thumped against me,
inside out,
And my heart skipped a beat,
Suddenly filled with doubt.

I waited and waited,
I begged you to come,
But you had other plans,
"Wait a little longer to be a mum."

My entire body ached
With the heaviness of your form
But your due date came and went,
And I awaited the storm.

I couldn't move,
It hurt too much,
I was sensitive to even
The tiniest touch.

I prayed to be safe.
I begged my body to lead,

But days came and passed,
And all I could do was plead.

Hands on my belly,
A pup at my feet,
But you weren't there yet.
I cried in defeat.

* * *

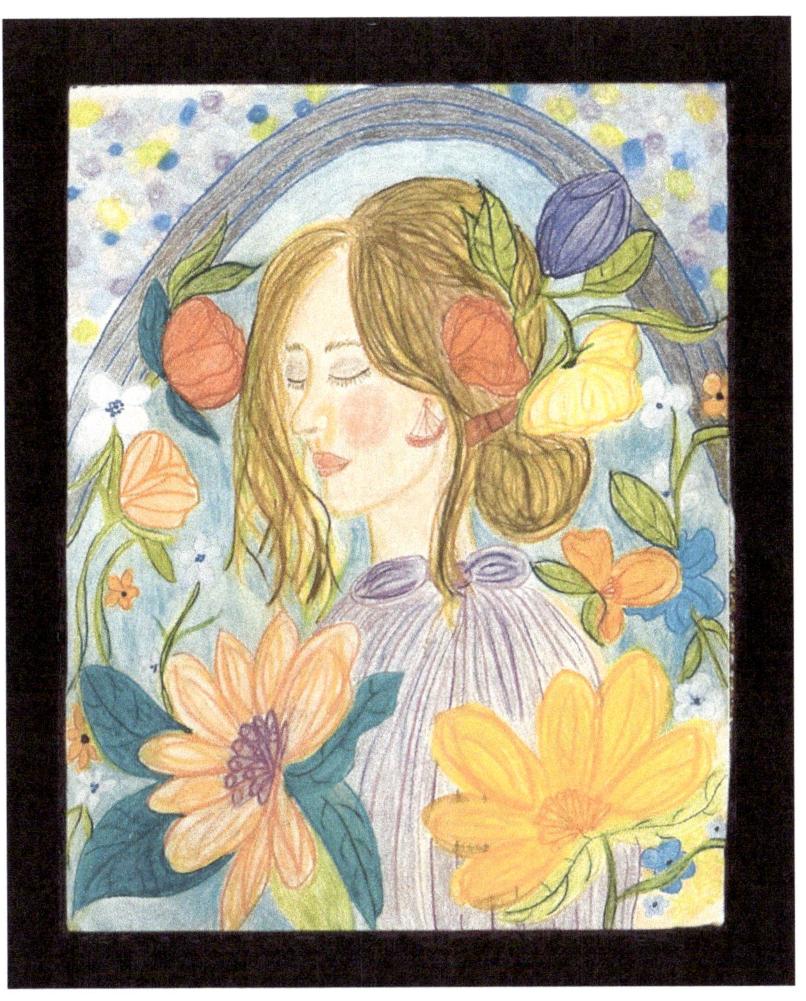

*"**Special**", Colored pencils, 2024*

Preparing and bearing

My body, scarred and marked,
Stretches with new wounds as the weeks pass,
My belly protruding to its limits,
It braces for what's to come.

Everything will change again
In this new season
Of small yet mighty cries and golden milk
And I won't recognize myself once more.

I'll look in the mirror
to see a visage peer back,
An empty, vacant shell of herself
Full of self doubt as a mother and wife.

Who is she, this woman pale with worry?
Her light has extinguished so.
I watch her fall from reality,
Back into the throes of familiar darkness.

Perhaps she'll surprise me,
Emerging, a Phoenix, into motherhood again,

But I fear she'll return to that lonesome world
Where grief and despair mingle.

I cannot bear the thought
Of her swift and sudden fall.
Yet I painfully brace myself,
Awaiting the collision.

If I forget in the hazy days to come,
I love my baby girl,
I promise, I do.
I just hope she knows that, too.

II

Birth

Hello, God?

I shook so violently, I thought I was dying.
I couldn't move, I couldn't speak, but I know I was crying.

The bright lights flashed above my eyes,
but I didn't know if I was alive.
They asked if I wanted to see you born,
but I was so tired, weak, and worn.

I couldn't breathe, I couldn't form words.
My voice could not be heard.

I panicked and called your name, but you weren't there.
And not a single person bothered to care.

The nausea rose and all I could say was, "Puke."
But they did nothing, just rebuke.

The sensations were awful, but I only got flashes,
of the way their scalpels were forming slashes.

I didn't hear your first cry…
I honestly just thought I was going to die.

I remember briefly giving you a kiss,
But the next five hours, I'd miss.

For months before, I repeated affirmations.
I thought I'd meet you with elation.

I told myself I was born to birth,
and when my body failed, I thought so did my worth.

I didn't die, but there were moments I wished I did,
because my pain and suffering, my sanity undid.

I couldn't even properly birth my own son,
In no way did it feel like I won.

"At least the baby's okay!" they say.
Maybe I will be... *some other day*.

* * *

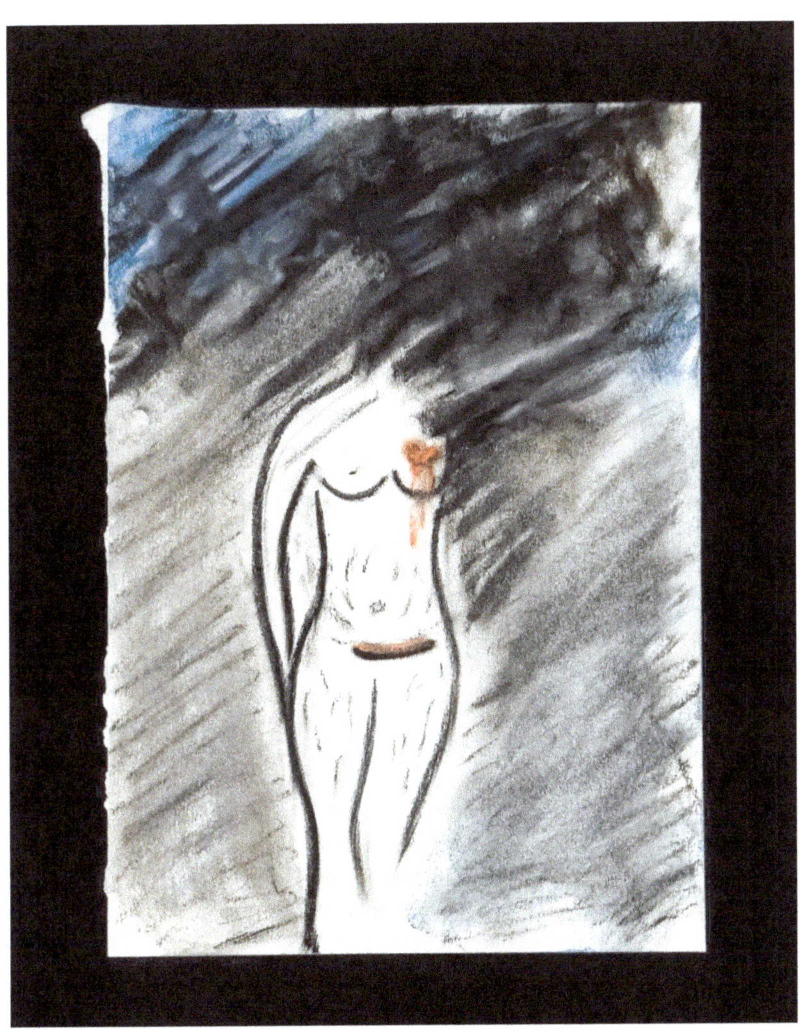

"Erasing in progress", Oil Pastels, 2019

Letter to the darkness

Dear Death,
I knocked upon your door,
And you answered quickly,
Inviting and pulling me in,
though I didn't know where I was,
And you lured me to the darkness,
To the bitter unknown,
And I almost gave up,
And let you take me,
Away from my baby,
Away from my family,
But even in the faint murmurings of my heart,
I knew I couldn't let go of the world,
And I slammed the door in your face,
I fought to survive.
Because I just…wasn't ready to die.

* * *

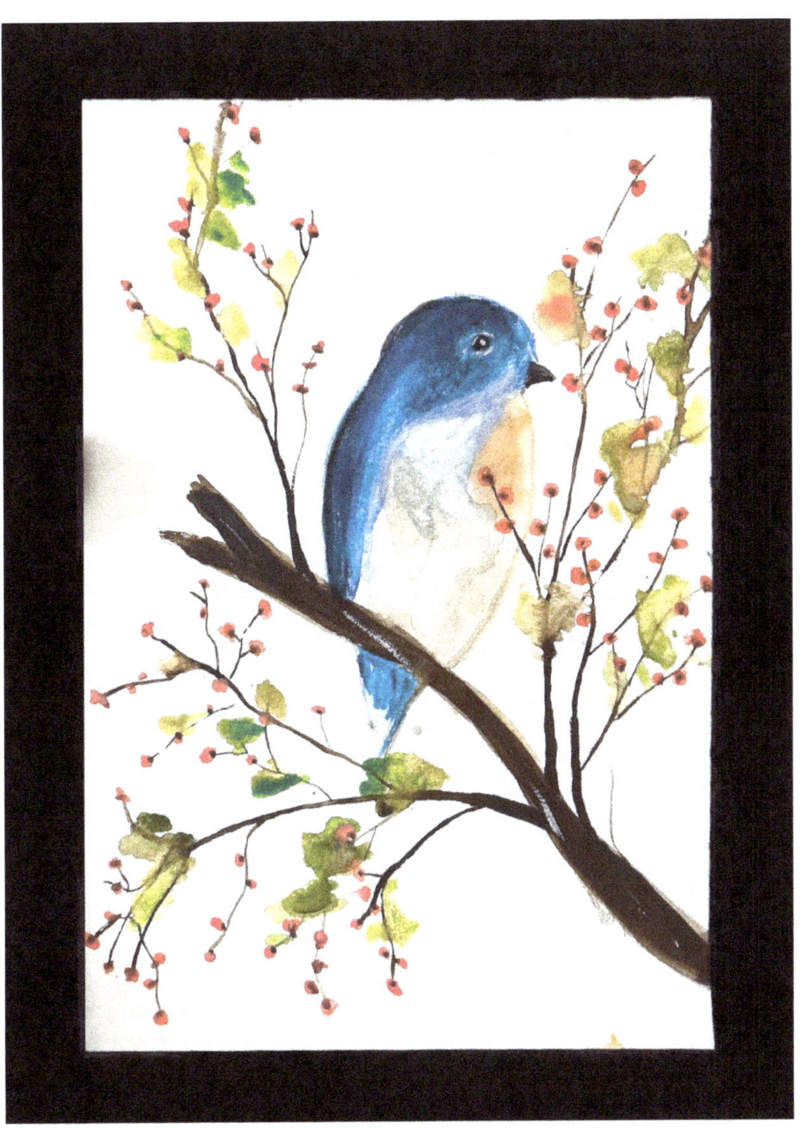

"Blue in Spring", *Watercolor, 2024*

Meeting…who?

I couldn't count your fingers or toes,
Because I couldn't wake up from below.

I saw a glimpse of you through heavy lidded eyes,
But then they closed, and I thought I died.

I took a picture with you in my bed,
But I don't recall, my body was lead.

Maybe you cried for me, I wish I knew…
But I just don't remember meeting you.

* * *

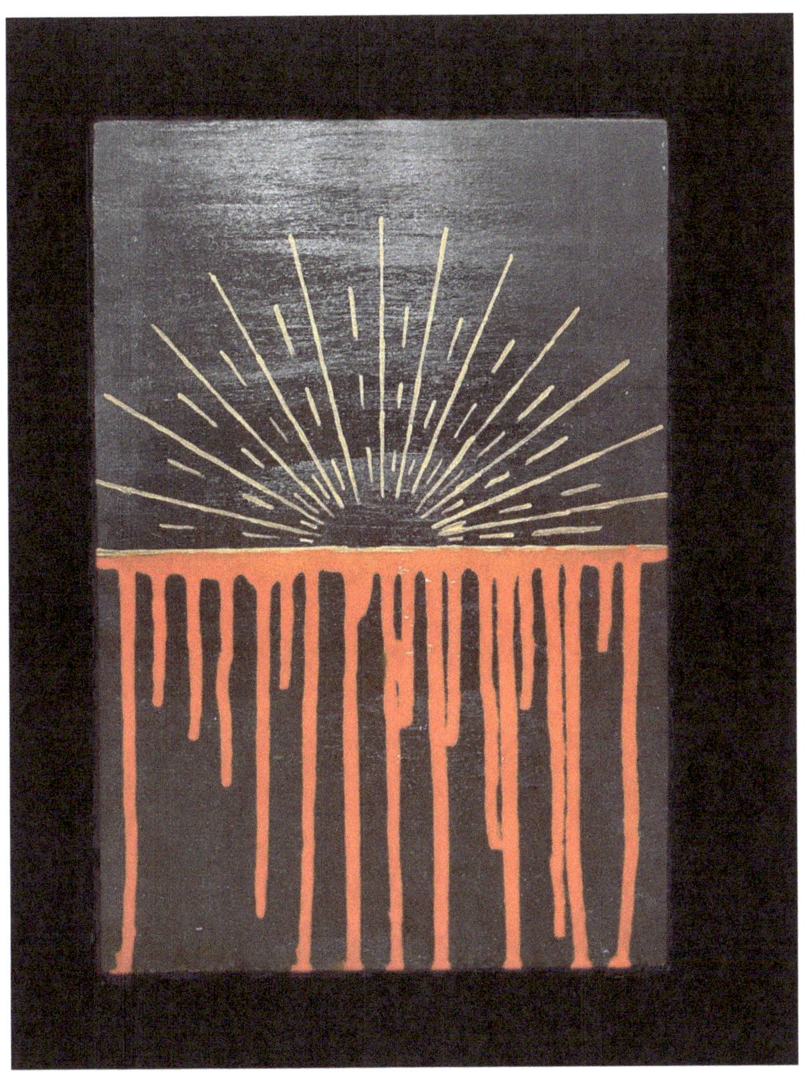

*"**I bleed for you**", Acrylic, 9" x 12", 2020*

Doom Day

The lullaby over the speaker jingled.
You asked me the date,
as if I was supposed to know.
Don't you know I almost died today?
I don't even know the year.

* * *

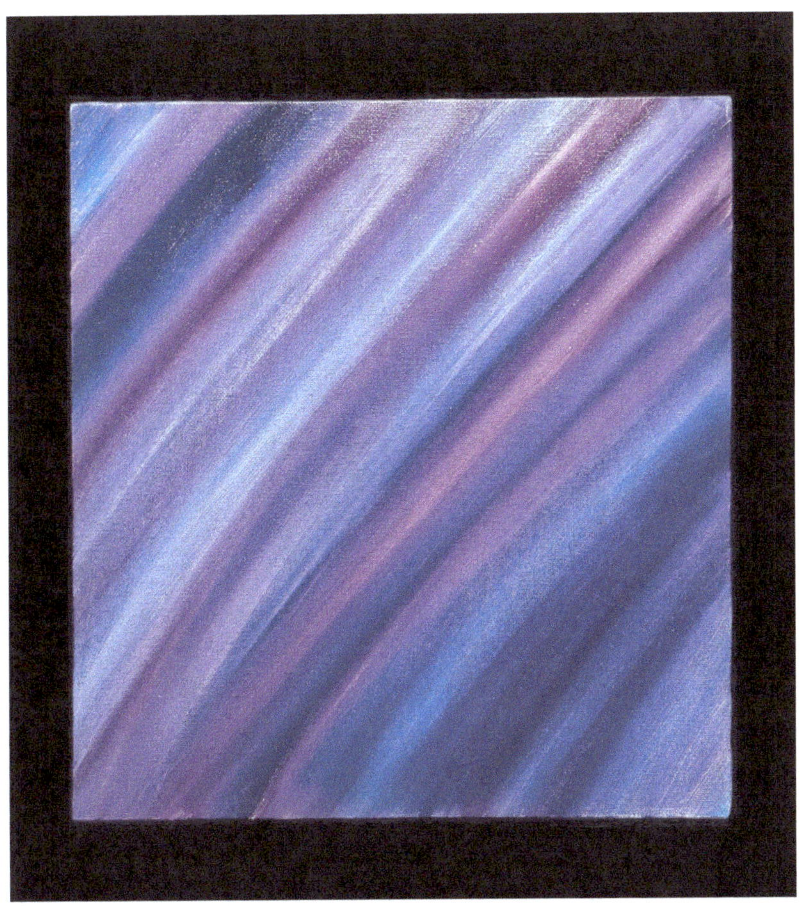

"Blue Slide", Oils, 12" x 12", 2022

Mad little mother

They thought I was crazy, they thought I was mad,
"Awe poor little mother, she just feels a bit bad,
She's fine, you know, just get her up,
Honestly, she can get her own cup.
Let her do it, she needs to learn how,
Oh, come on, what now?"

"You don't need help to get in the shower."
It had been more than 96 hours…
I begged for someone to bring me to pee,
But apparently the burden was too weighty.

Baby wouldn't latch, but nobody would come,
They simply acted like I was dumb.
The cut off my meds without a word,
Then scoffed as my eyes in pain blurred.
My baby was ten and half pounds,
Yet they couldn't make time for me in their rounds.

Only one nurse finally showed me some kindness,
Apologizing for the others' blindness.
She told me she'd never seen anyone else go through,

Everything I had been trying to subdue.

She was the only saving grace in that whole awful place,
I don't remember much, but I'll always remember her face.

* * *

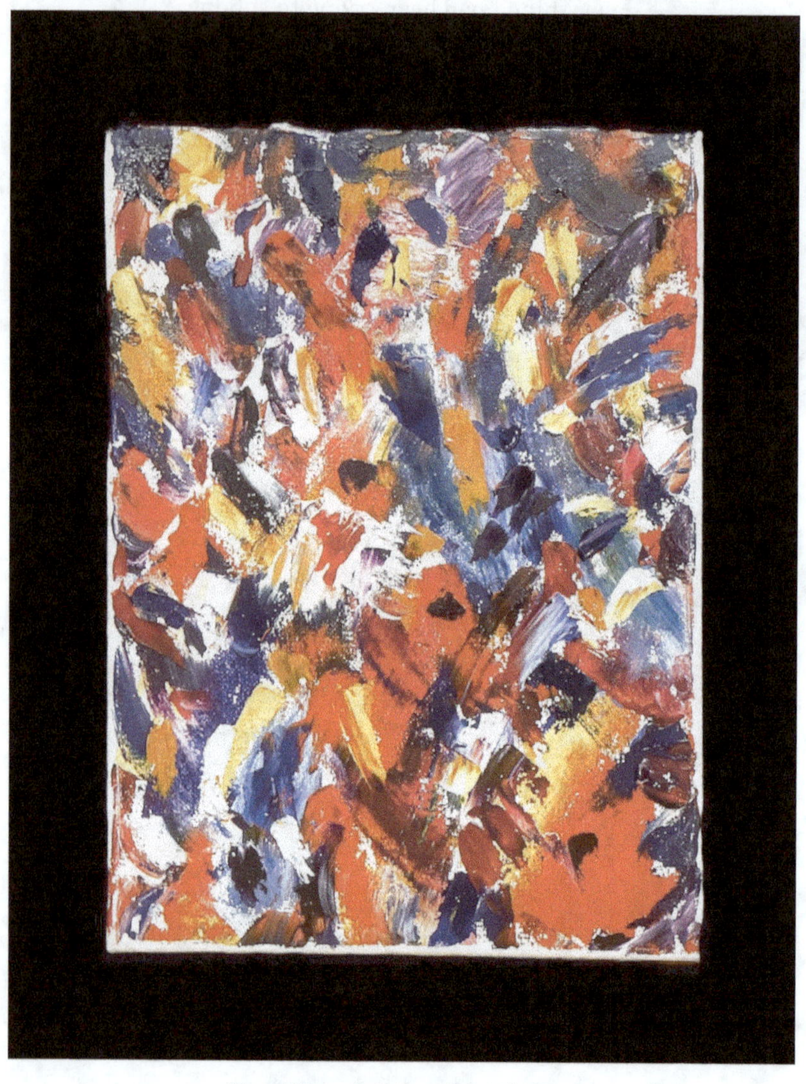

"Set Ablaze", Oils, 8" x 10", 2022

The barrage

"Let's get you up,
You can't sit in bed,
No need to be dramatic,
The pain is just in your head.

The baby's fine,
Be grateful you didn't die,
Get over it,
You gave it a try.

Twenty more doctors
Will visit you today,
They will swarm your room,
No, you don't get a say.

Breast is best,
He needs to constantly feed,
Formula is simply awful,
We'll make you plead.

You seriously don't know
The date today?

Come on,
Let's get you weighed.

You don't need any meds,
You'll just get hooked,
Honestly, it's a crutch,
But your sepsis we overlooked.

We don't buy
That everything's completely hazy,
Instead we'd rather believe,
You're just a little crazy.

Go home, it's fine,
There's nothing we can do,
You're still sick and broken,
But now it's on you."

* * *

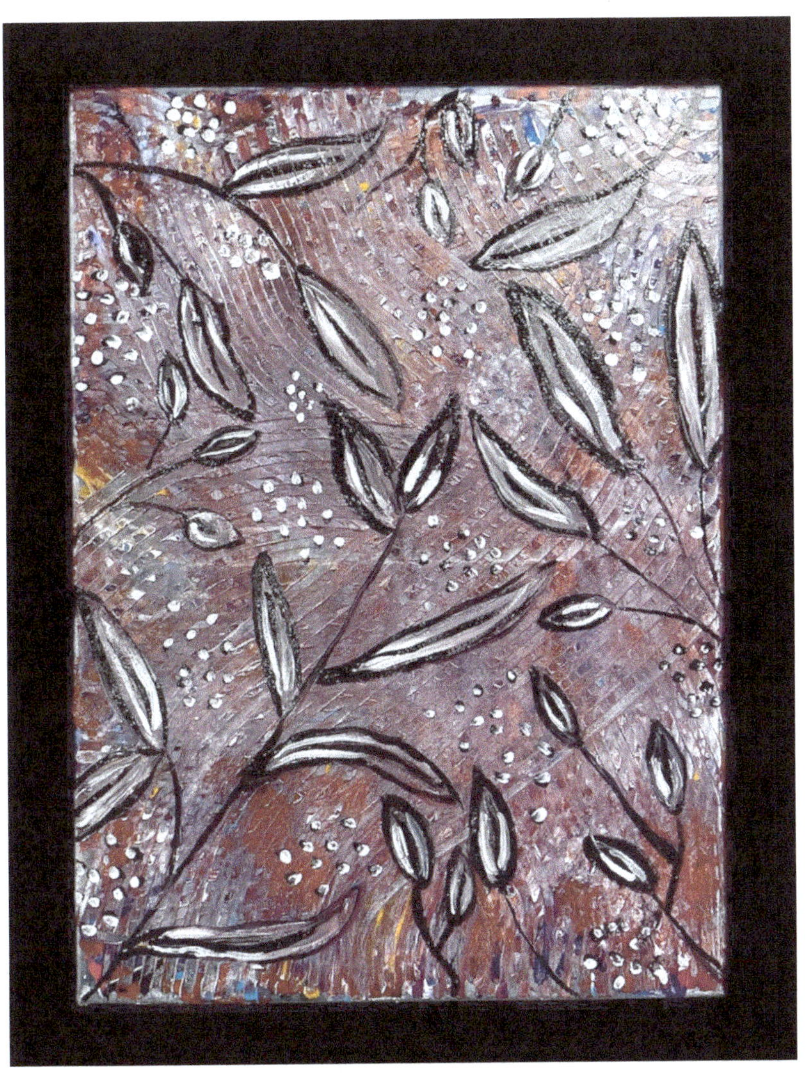

*"**Growth**", Acrylic, 18" x 24", 2023*

III

So New, Me and You

A wish come due

Home from the hospital, home with you,
I feel like it's the first time I've had a view,
To look at you and count your toes,
To wonder at your button nose.

You're curled up against my chest,
And for a moment, I think, "This is the best."
You're finally here, we survived after all,
Maybe God really did answer my call.

* * *

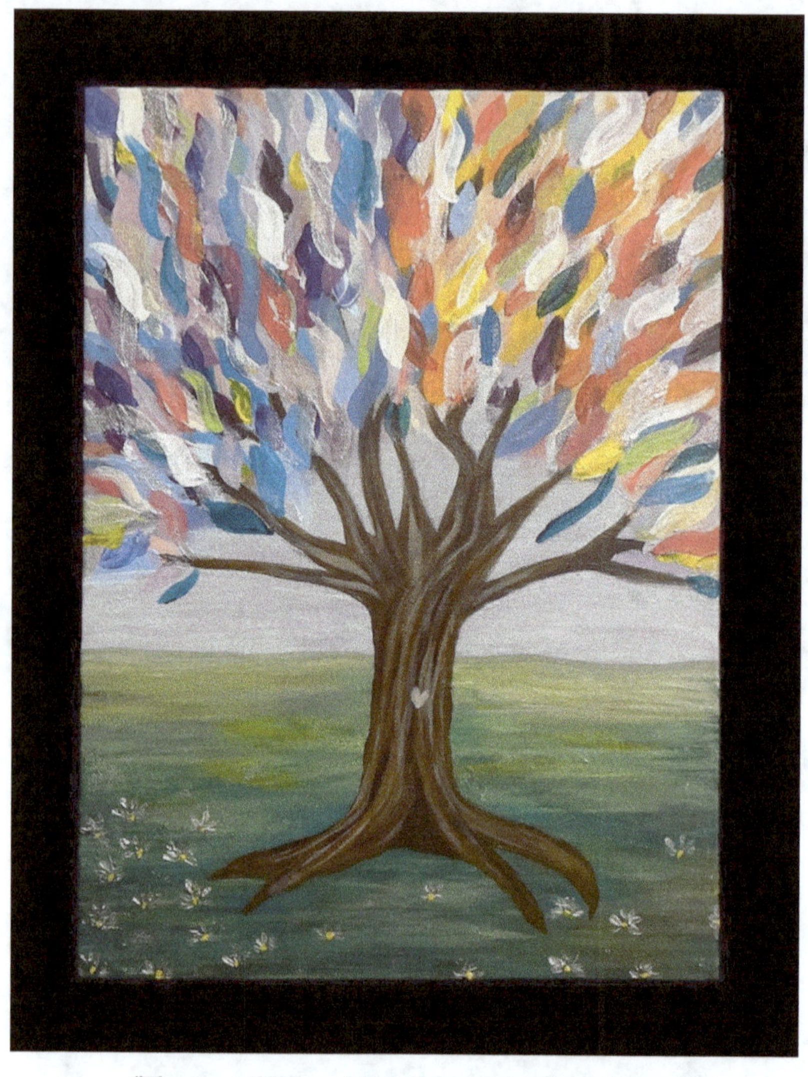

"The tree of life and love", Acrylic, 12" x 16", 2023

Full Arms

I couldn't set you down,
Not even for a second,
Even though I struggled deeply,
Your cries persistently beckoned.

I held you close
Against my chest,
Allowing us both
To finally rest.

I carried you with me
Throughout the day,
And you slept on me restlessly,
Me sometimes wishing it away.

But I wanted you close,
I almost lost you once,
And the panic remained,
Even after months.

I rocked you to sleep,
A bad habit I was told,

But nothing was more important,
Than you in my arms to hold.

Stranger Danger

I was convinced he wasn't mine,
Because I didn't see his birth.
I feared he had to be for someone else,
Because he was a stranger to me.
This baby I had grown for 42 weeks,
Didn't even look like my son,
Because I couldn't make my brain believe he was mine.
I wasted a year of my life trying to shake that belief.
All that time… I couldn't connect,
Even though I loved him so much.
But who was he?
If I didn't see it happen, did I even give birth?
Or was it just some sick twisted nightmare?

* * *

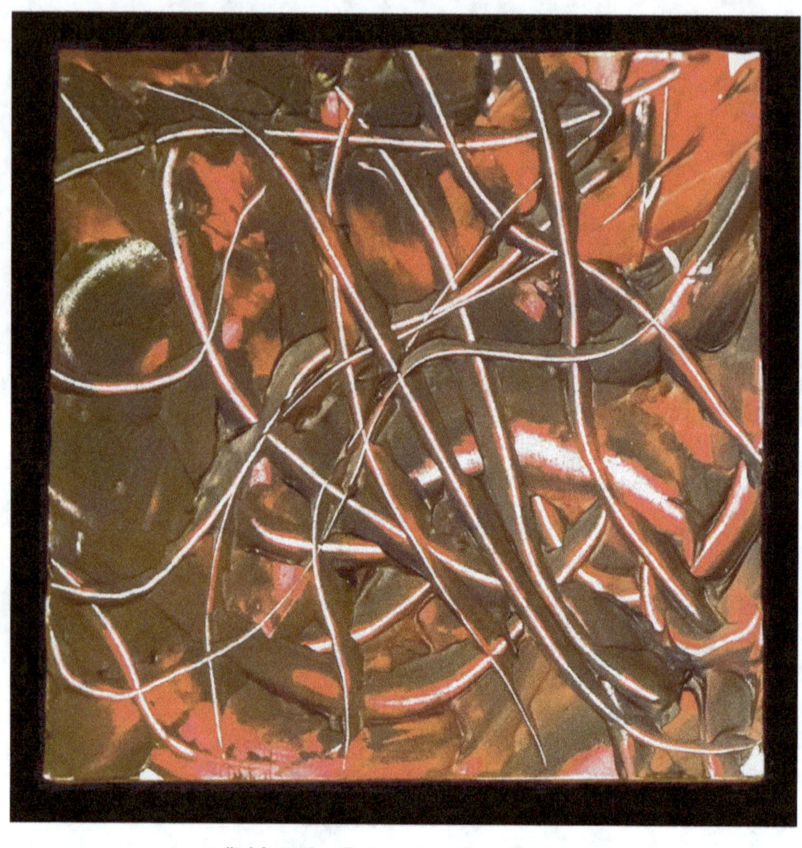

*"**Life Wire**", Acrylic, 6" x 6", 2020*

New

The baby was okay.
I suppose so was I.
I was told I should be grateful.
After all, I didn't die.
I guess I should be happy.
But instead I'm filled with grief.
There are no more chances
Nor do I want there to be,
I wish it could have been different.
I'm allowed to deeply mourn,
Even as I hold this precious gift
Safe in my arms.

* * *

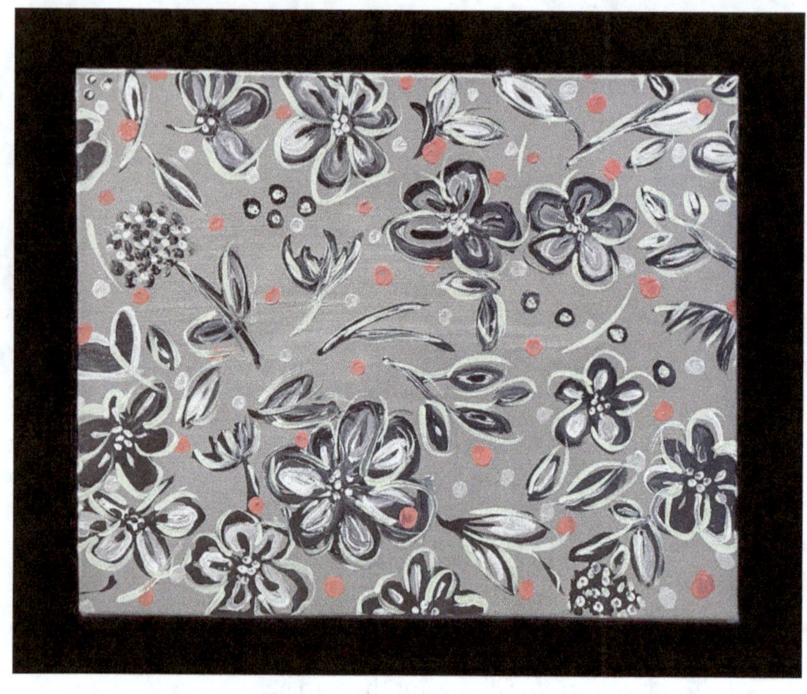

*"**Refresh**", Acrylic, 16" x 20" , 2023*

Returning Away and Coming Back to You

I pull on the jeans that barely fit
Over my swollen belly and soft hips.

I put on makeup, some foundation maybe,
Is this the first time since the baby?

I'm returning to work because I must,
But am I losing my child's trust?

A few short weeks we had together
And now I'm forced away, a day feels like forever.

Focus on work while my body still bleeds,
I can't focus...I won't succeed.

I count the hours, the clock ticks slow,
But my true emotions I cannot show.

The clock strikes five. I race home.
Sweet baby, I'm so sorry I left you alone.

Forgive me please, I love you so.

I just wish I didn't have to go.

* * *

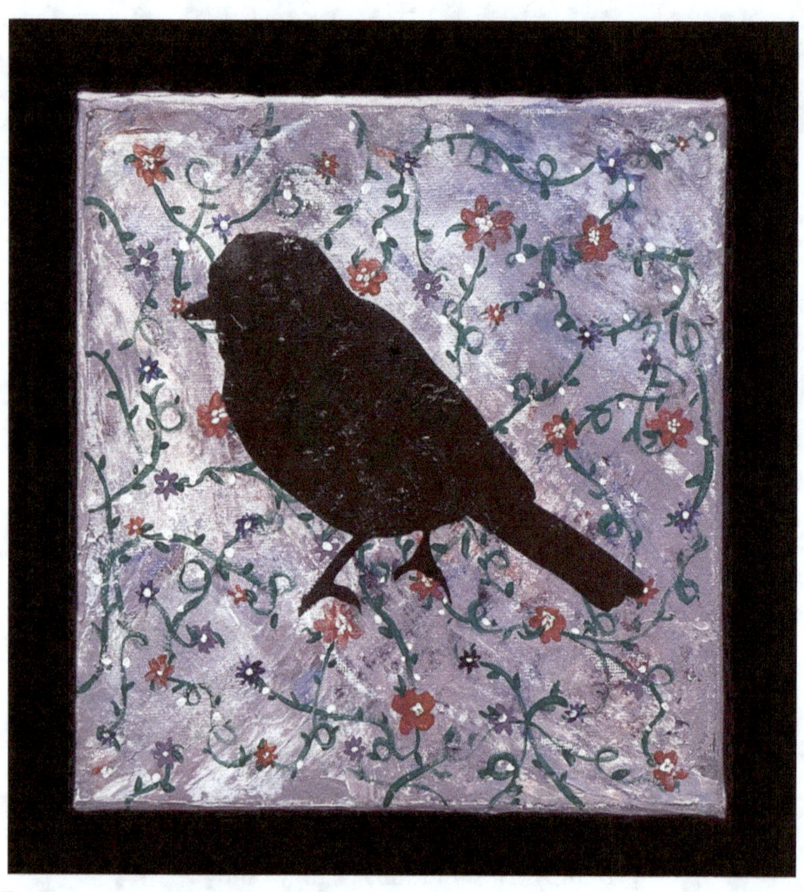

"The Song Bird", Acrylic, 8" x 8", 2020

Breast to Depressed

I bring you to my chest, such a natural thing to do,
But it doesn't feel okay, for either of us it seems.
I feel sick, I feel like I'll vomit.
And you seem angry…like you can't get enough.
I try and try to feed you with my body,
the way it's intended to do,
And I send myself into depression
about the few drops I get,
Because my body is supposed to work.
And it failed you in birth,
And now it can't even feed you.
"Breast is best", but why can't I do it?
I must be a failure.
I was supposed to be able to do this for my baby.
Am I a bad mom if I have to give him formula?
I guess I'll try until my mental health is shot.
I didn't know it was okay to stop.

Overwhelm at the Helm

The dishes piled up again,
The bottles scattered across the den.

And the guilt ate at me, more than I could bear,
Did I change my underwear?

The laundry towered in a heap,
When was the last time I found sleep?

I constantly nursed, pumped and burped a back,
But I could never seem to eat a snack.

Dinner came from a box again,
I hadn't showered, I didn't remember when.

Why was this so hard to do?
I swore I didn't have a clue.

But then I looked at you and smiled,
As you held my finger for a while.

And I finally decided, this was another day's fight.

OVERWHELM AT THE HELM

Looking at you, I guessed I was doing something right.

* * *

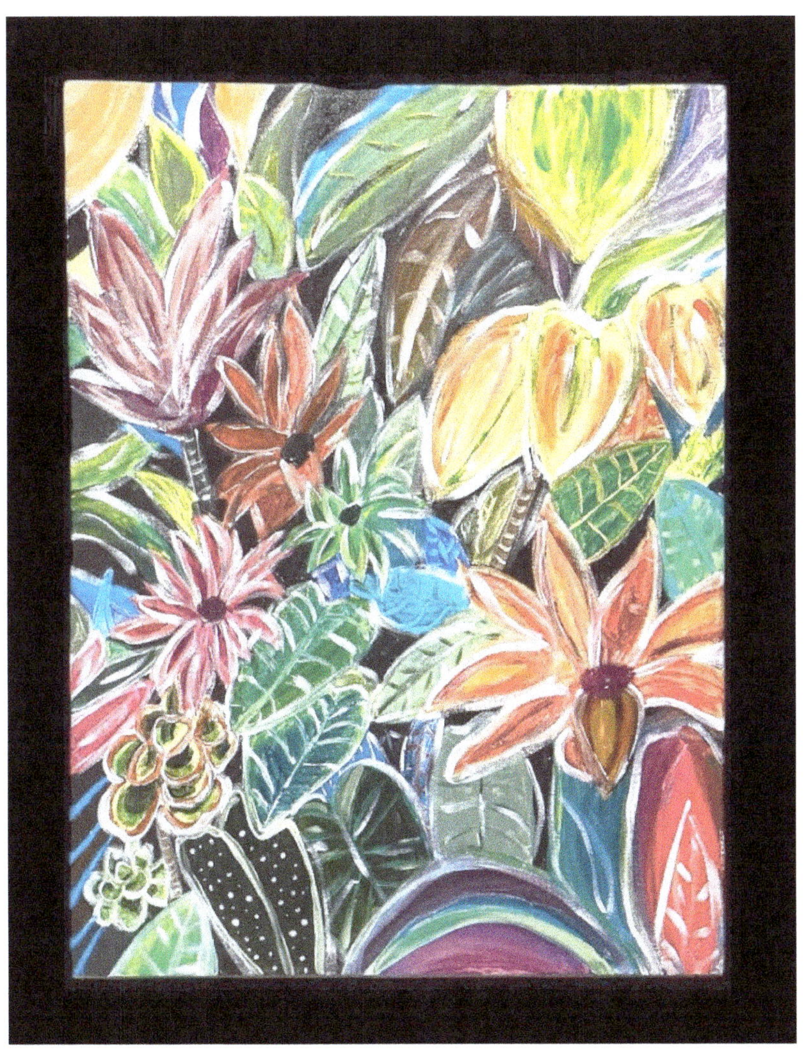

"Lost in the jungle", Acrylic, 16" x 20", 2023

Drip, Drop, Kerplop

That precious golden milk is gone.
I weep as I see the dawn.

A drip,
a drop,
a spill…
kerplop.

I watch it crash to the floor,
Because I bumped into the door.

"Don't cry over spilled milk," you say,
But my nipples were the ones who had to pay.

You don't understand the load
Of feeling your breasts might implode.

"Please, please just stop…
I pumped an hour to fill that to the top."

* * *

"Cotton Candy Sky", Acrylic, 6" x 6", 2022

Once and Twice

Rock you once, rock you twice,
Swaddled and warm and snug and tight.
Pace the room once, pace the room twice,
Sing you a lullaby, it's so late at night.

Feed you once, change you twice,
Will you ever go to sleep, sweet baby?
You cry once, I cry twice,
We'll get a hang of this, maybe…

Your eyes close once, mine close twice,
But I can't lay you down.
I shush once, I pat twice,
I must be the only one up in town.

He snores once, I sob twice,
I've never been this alone.
Deep breath once, swallow twice,
You're still a stranger I've grown.

Close Alarm

I almost set the house on fire,
Because I was so damn tired.

And all I could hear were your screams in my ear.
Nobody but you and me were here.

But you wouldn't stop, and I couldn't help.
I'd hold you and you'd just yelp.

I paced the house with you in my arms,
Until I finally heard the alarms.

There was smoke everywhere, gray and thick.
I forgot it in the microwave…your screams in an uptick.

Nothing helped. You never slept.
We both just constantly wept.

And I couldn't seem to figure out why,
Why, baby, why did you cry?

Colic? Gas? What did you need?

Your screaming picked up speed.

I thought I was going crazy, I thought I was going wild.
Why did nobody tell me it would be this way with a child?

* * *

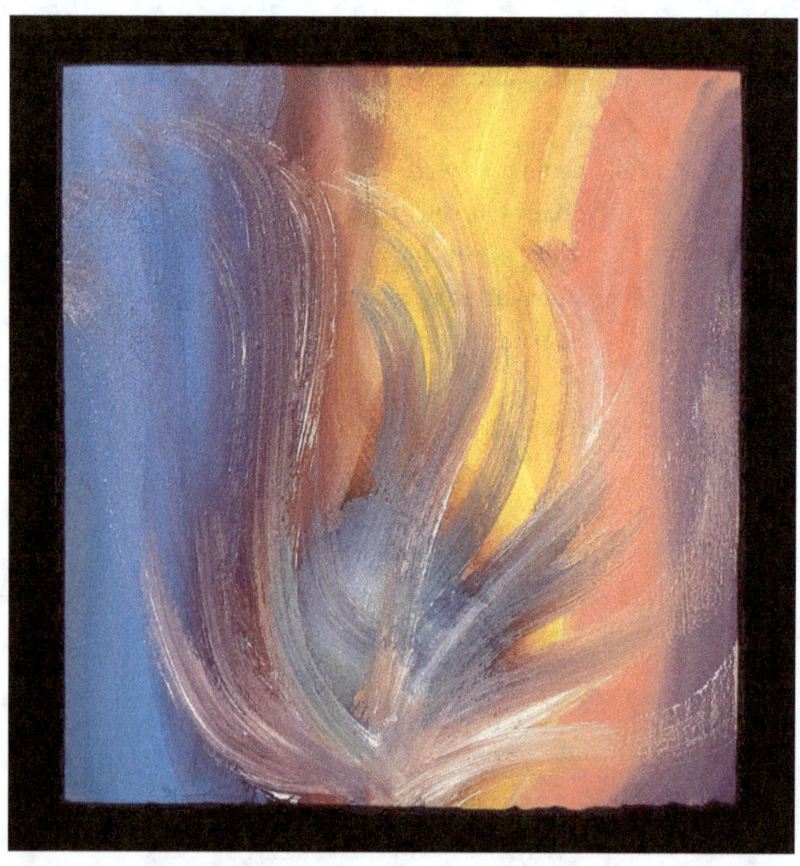

"The Light From Within", Acrylic, 7" x 7", 2021

High Needs, My Ear Bleeds

You wail, and scream, and I'm beside myself,
I lean heavily against the bookshelf.

I see a tear form in your eye,
And now I, too, begin to cry.

Who's turn is it to wail, is it yours or mine?
"Yes, I swear I'm fine!"

I don't know you, I don't recognize me,
Yet somehow we're supposed to be a "we".

I haven't showered in days it seems,
I just want to feel the water stream.

But I can't leave you, or you'll cry,
And I swear, that makes me want to die.

Where is my village? Where is my tribe?
I'm just lucky to be alive.

I'm healing, bleeding, sore, and in pain,

And to myself I place all the shame and blame.

Maybe I wasn't meant to be a mom,
If I can't even make my baby calm.

Who's crying? Is it your turn or mine?
Screw it… I'm not…fine.

* * *

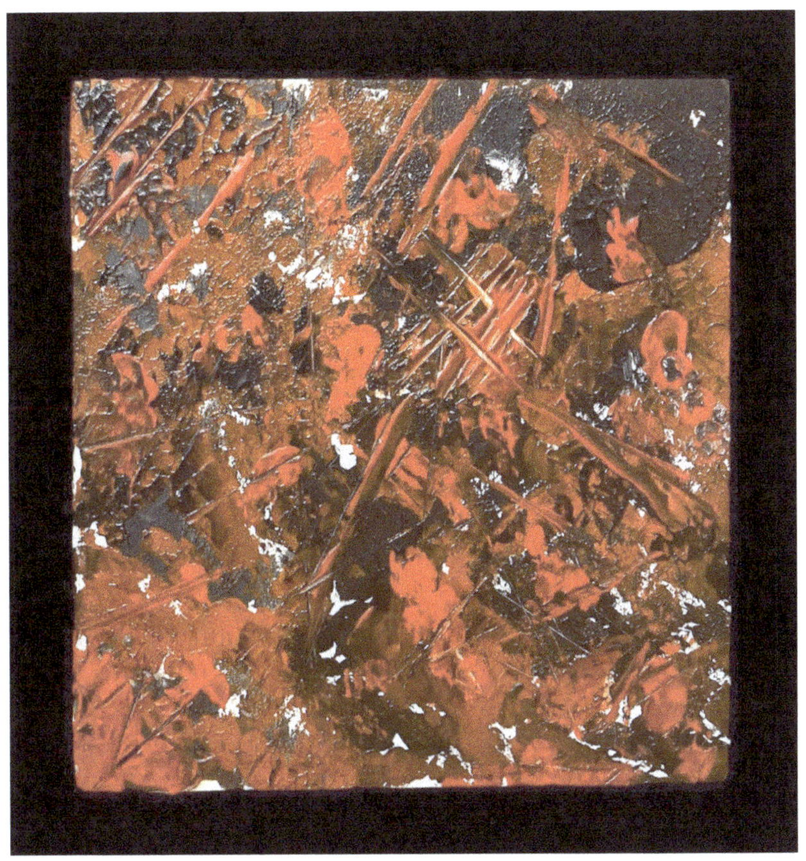

*"**Inside My Veins**", Acrylic, 6" x 6", 2020*

IV

Drowning

An Unexpected Rage

An ugly venom built inside.
I'm angry, so angry!, "But it's fine," I lied.

But then a little thing would make me burst,
And every day I felt my worst.

I couldn't see up from down,
All I could see was my hatred around,

For those who didn't lift a finger,
For the baby vomit smell that lingered.

I felt a hurricane of rage,
Because postpartum felt like a cage.

And every day I felt myself snap,
Trying to soothe the baby on my lap.

And nobody knew why I was so mad,
But really deep inside, I was just so sad.

I couldn't explain it, I didn't know how,

Those feelings I couldn't myself allow.

For if I did, the worst mom I'd be.
Someone who desperately wanted to be free,
Of the shackles of motherhood, of the chains of time,
Of spousal priorities that no longer aligned.

Nobody seemed to understand,
My deliberate writing in the sand.

Mental health after birth is no joke,
But the hold on your life can make you choke.

* * *

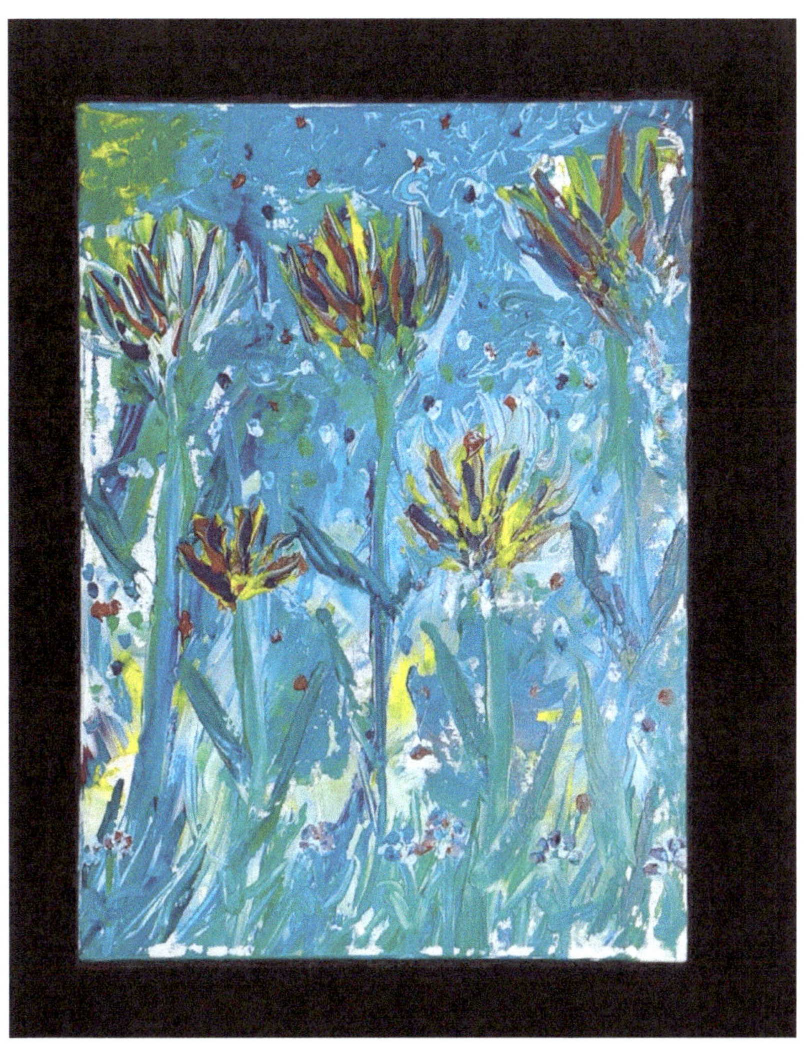

"Growing Through Despair", Acrylic, 16" x 20", 2023

Dragging the Darkness

For some who graze death's hand
They find a desire to live
But I was consumed with the fear to die.
If it could nearly happen on a Saturday morning,
What's to say it wouldn't come again for me
On a Wednesday night while I slept?
Or on a Monday afternoon while the baby played?
My light almost went out,
And the darkness suffocated me.

* * *

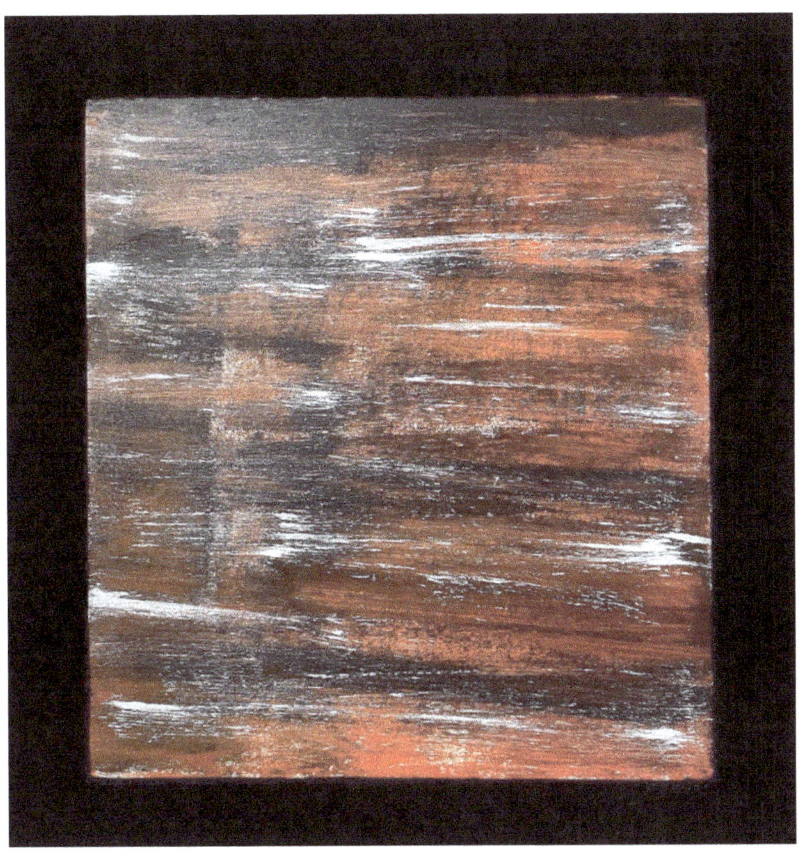

*"**Static**", Acrylic, 6" x 6", 2022*

What's That Noise?

I heard her cry, I *swear* I did,
Something awful is going to happen.
Will I drop her, will she *die*?
Will she *choke* on the blankie satin?

The milk's too hot, it will *burn* her mouth,
She's too cold, she'll surely get *sick*.
Did I leave the *stove* on, is the door locked?
My mind is playing every trick.

I don't set her down,
Because what if she *falls*?
I *panic* in circles,
What if there's *mold* in the walls?

I'm *crawling* out of my skin, I swear,
I am *terrified* it will all go wrong.
What's that you say? I'm not *crazy* at all?
I guess it was postpartum *anxiety* all along.

* * *

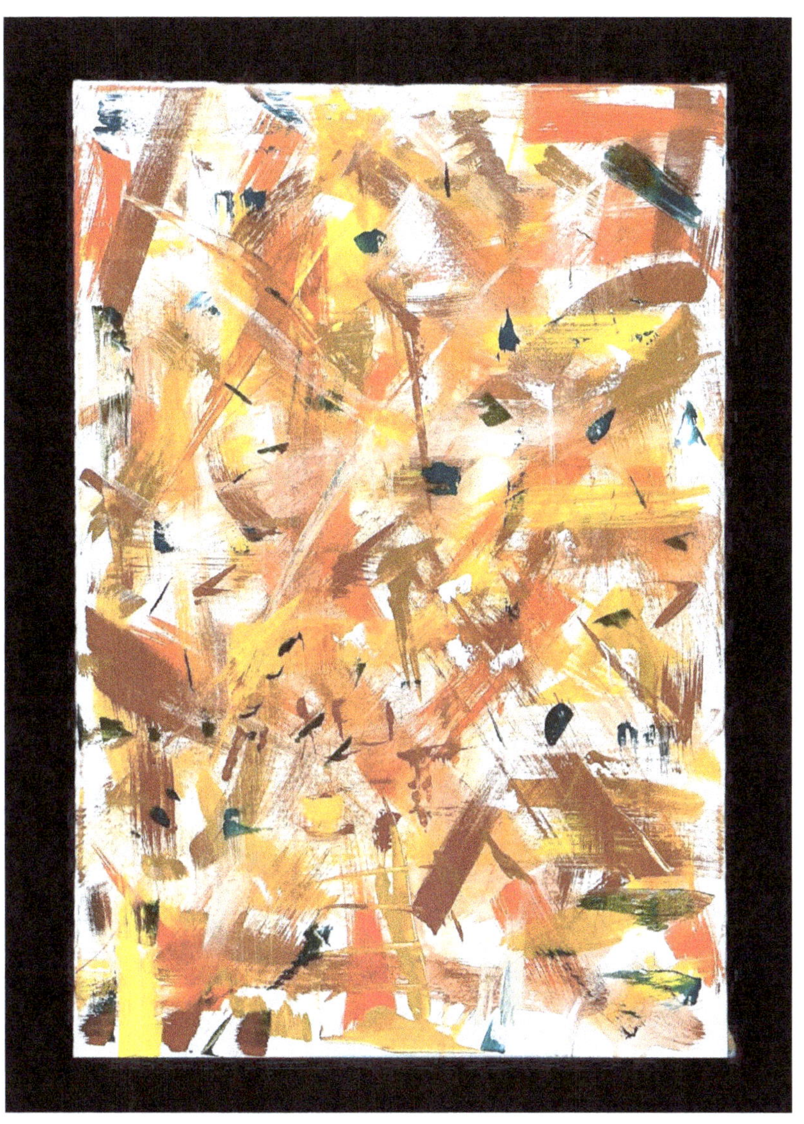

"Reclaimed", Acrylic, 18" x 24", 2023

I'm Still Here

Please…
witness me.
In my grief.
In my pain.
In my vulnerability.
Witness me,
and don't run away.

* * *

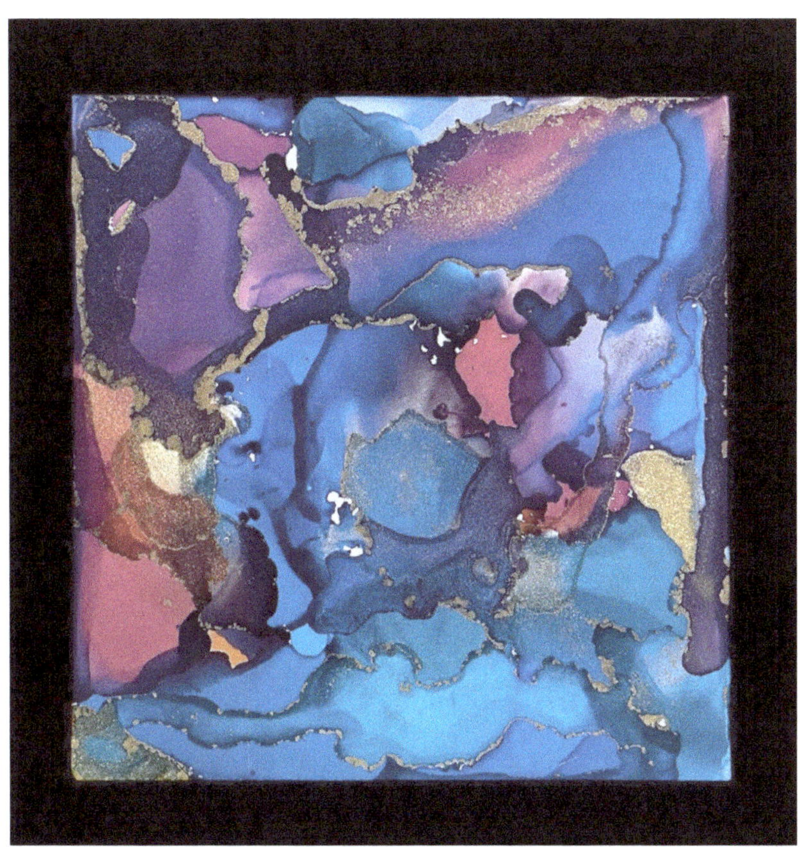

"Precious Jewels", Alcohol Inks, 4" x 4", 2019

Roar

Pacing the same stretch
Over and over.
Clawing to get out.
I am eternally trapped
by my own mind.
I've become a wild caged animal.
I can't escape.
Will I ever be free?

* * *

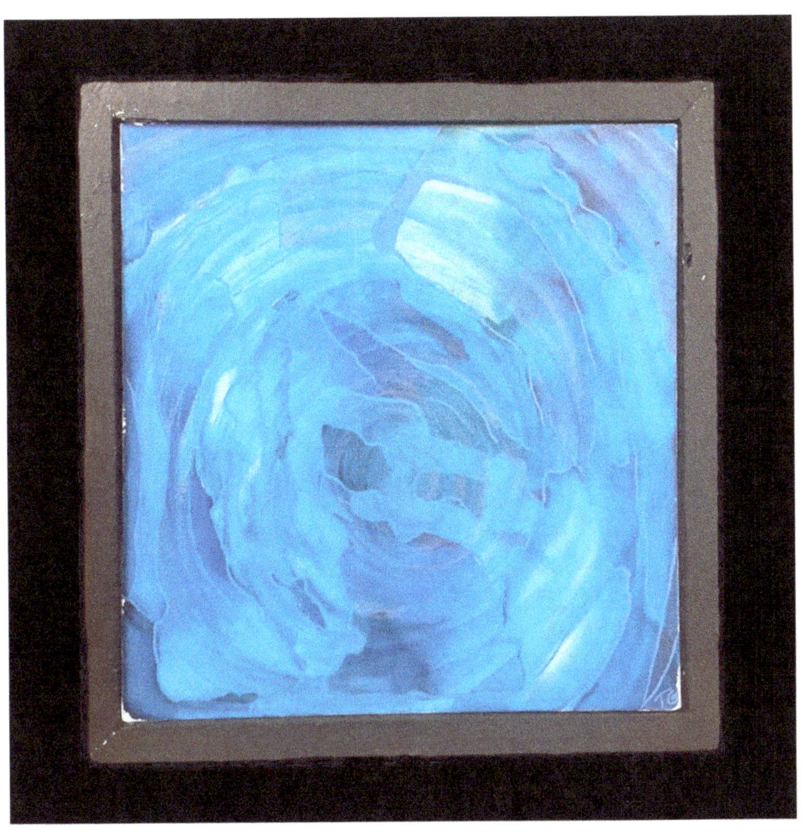

"The Mind Labyrinth", Alcohol Inks, 6" x 6", 2021

Infested

My grief is a weed
and there's an infestation
wrapped around my soul.

* * *

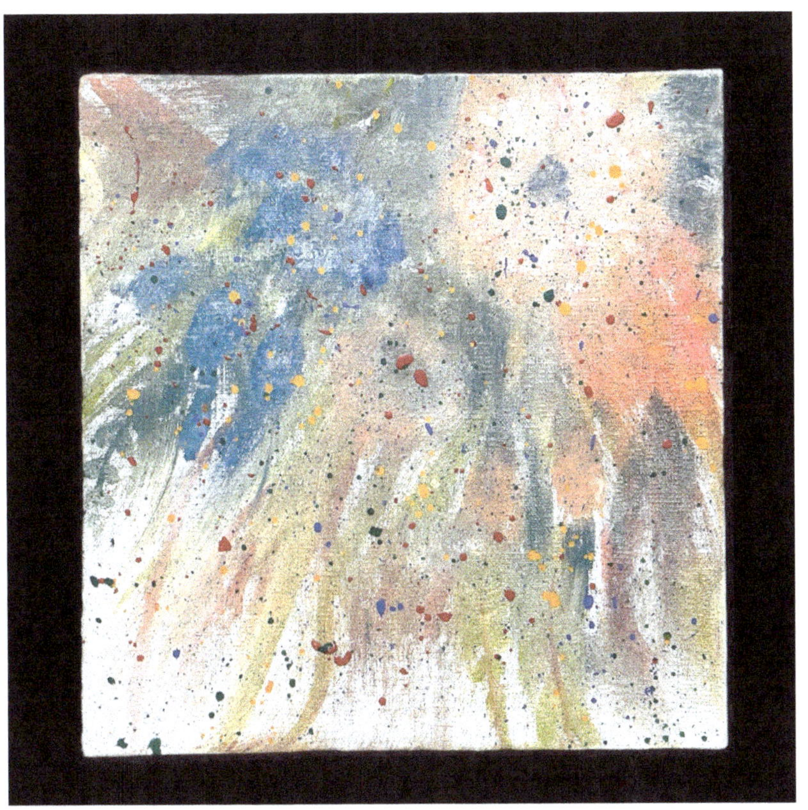

"I Can't See the Garden", Oils, 8" x 8", 2021

A World Unbothered While She Panics

Angst reverberated around her hollowness,
Threatening to rip apart the tattered seams,
Those which barely held her together.

A persistent rumbling of unease
settled over her in a fine dust,
One unable to be scrubbed from her skin.

She was all too familiar with these feelings.
They were long acquaintances,
But she wondered if there'd ever be reprieve.

Her view of the world had become skewed,
Unable to see any light,
through the thick veil of unending panic.

She sensed impending danger,
A feeling of doom lingered persistently,
Yet the rest of the world seemed unbothered.

She wondered if she'd ever feel safe again,
Out in public, at home, in her own body …

But that was a luxury she no longer possessed.

Peace was gone.
Tranquility and security a distant dream,
Shreds of hope left in its remains.

Sometimes the world breaks you,
Taking the most vital pieces of yourself
And leaving them for dead.

And what can you do
Except try to find life
In the shell of your old self?

* * *

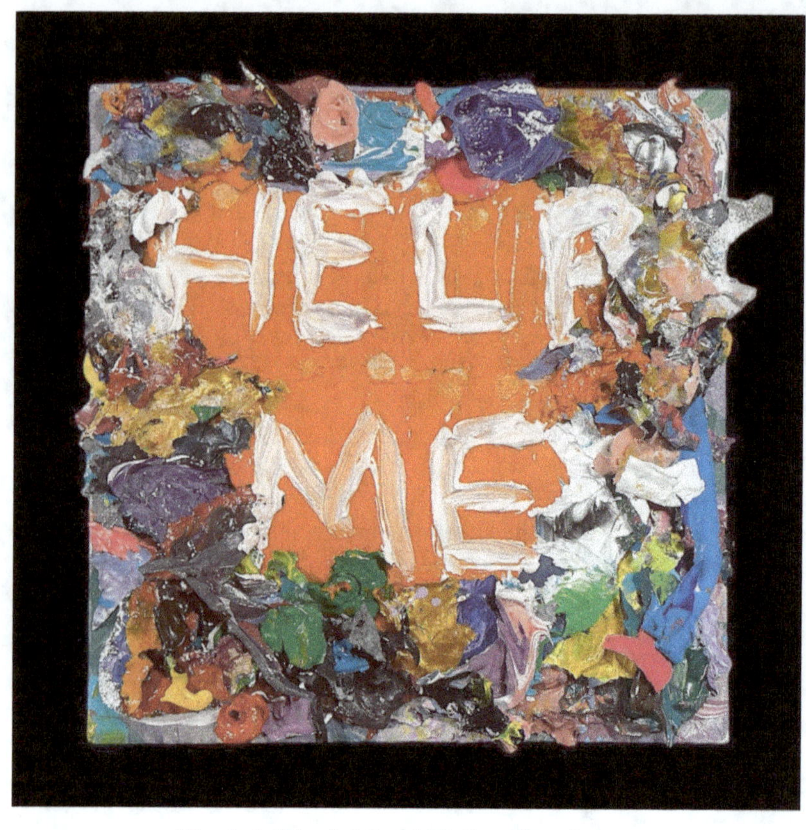

"Buried Alive", Mixed Media, 8" x 8", 2024

She Smiles

She bleeds.
Black and blue,
Her raw wounds pulse
With the loneliness
Of a thousand vacant skies.

She bleeds.
Her demons rally,
Clutching at her newly barren body,
Pulling her to the ground,
Covering every inch of her,
In shame and anger.

She bleeds.
Her bones are fragile,
Unable to hold the unbearable weight,
Of the impenetrable, deafening darkness
That looms around her,
Engulfing her in a joyless cocoon.

She bleeds.
The fear of unattainable worthiness

Squeezing tightly around her
As she holds her precious gift
In her longing arms
Knowing she may never be enough.

She bleeds.
Unlawful scars cover her flesh.
They crawl wildly across her body
As a constant reminder
Of her ultimate failure
In her first true act as a mother.

She bleeds.
And bleeds.
And bleeds.
Blood of regret.
Blood of sorrow.
Blood of heartache.

She bleeds.
But she smiles….
And the world forgets.

* * *

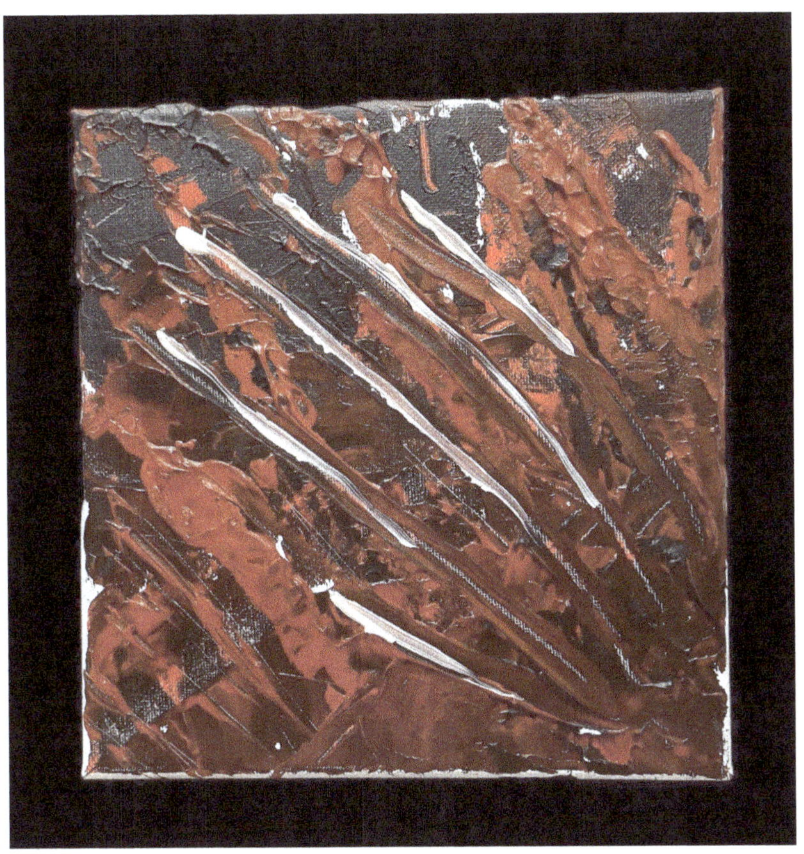

*"**Death's Grip**", Acrylic, 8" x 8", 2020*

Reminisce and Repeat

I was splayed open
to bring new life
While I hovered dangerously
on the brink of death.

And now I have to do it
all over again
And all I want to do is
turn and run.

Haven't I been cut open
and on display
enough in my life?

I Wonder Which

I don't know which is worse:
the *depth* of the darkness
or the *breadth* of the heartache.

* * *

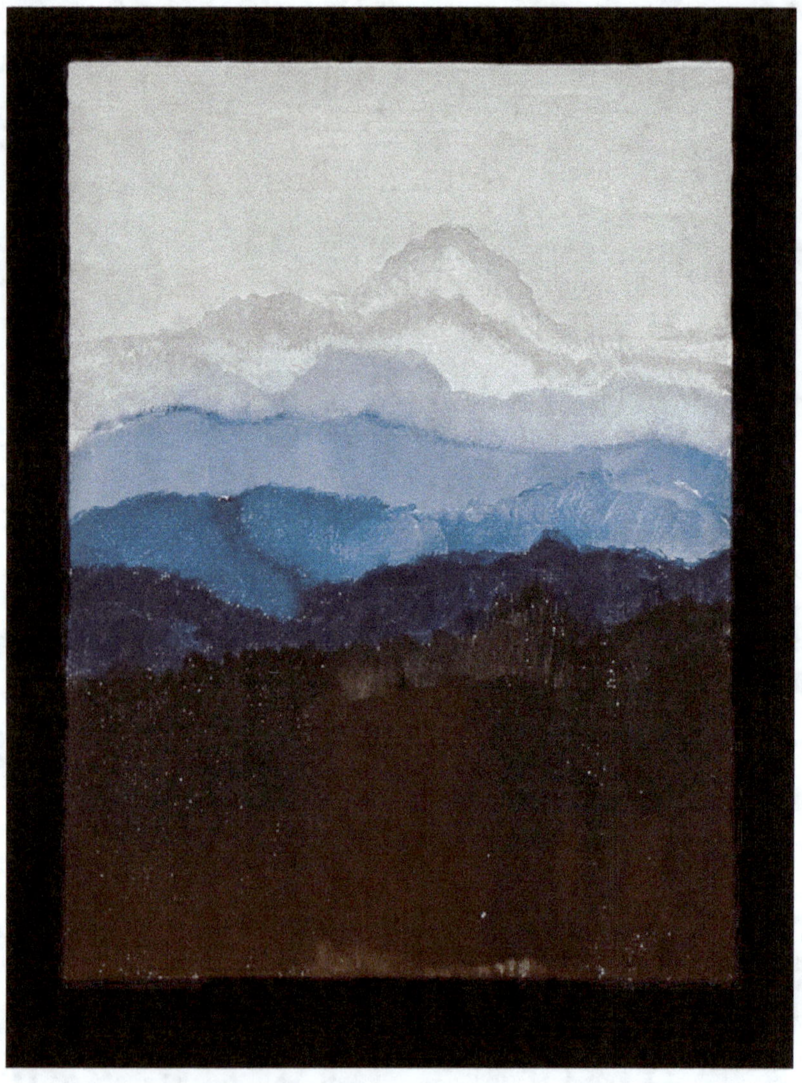

"Grief in the Mountains", Acrylic, 9" x 12", 2022

Maternal Mountain

I never
expected
motherhood to feel
like complete suffocation,
but here I am, trapped by the mountain
of unwavering responsibility,
and I can't catch
my breath
anymore.

* * *

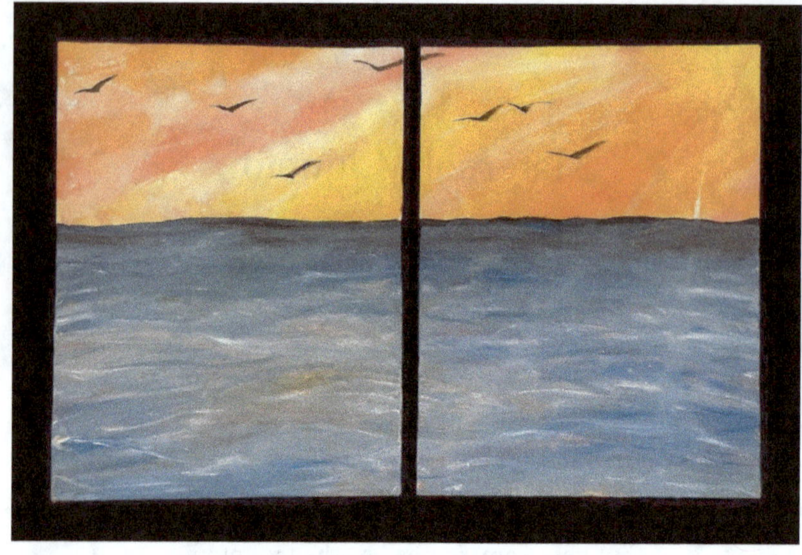

*"**Hovering**", Oils, two 16" x 20" panels, 2023*

Empty Forever

The enormity of loneliness
Engulfs me entirely
Not from the act of being alone
But rather the feeling
That I'll never feel
Whole again.

* * *

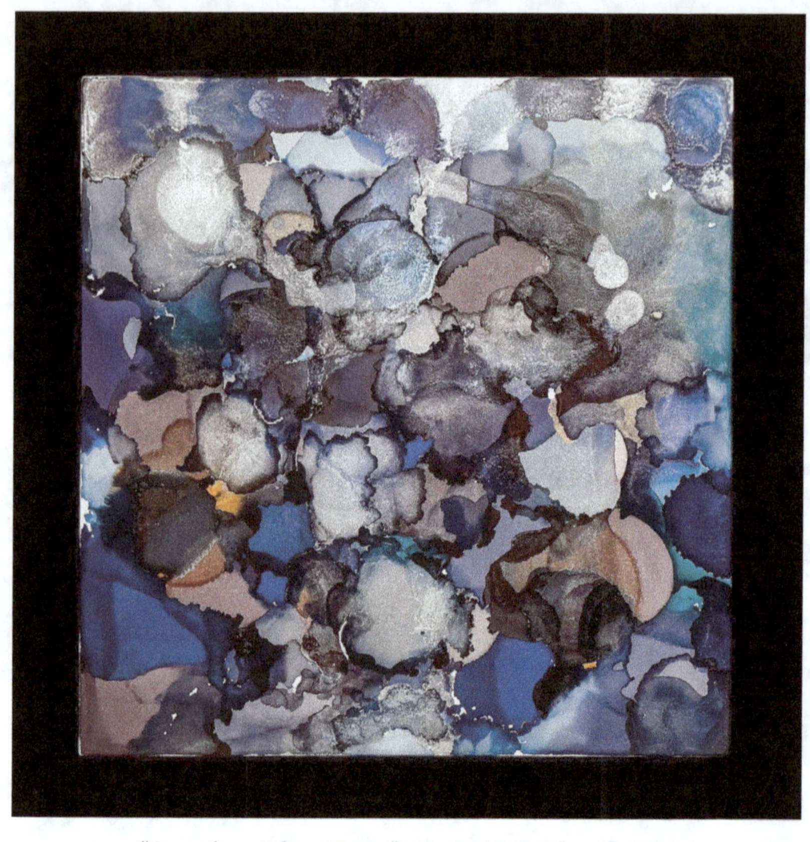

"Once in a Blue Moon", Alcohol Ink, 6" x 6", 2021

Black Lace

The darkness surrounds me,
and laces its fingers between mine.
I seek an elusive light that never comes.
And so we become inescapable companions,
Me and the darkness.

* * *

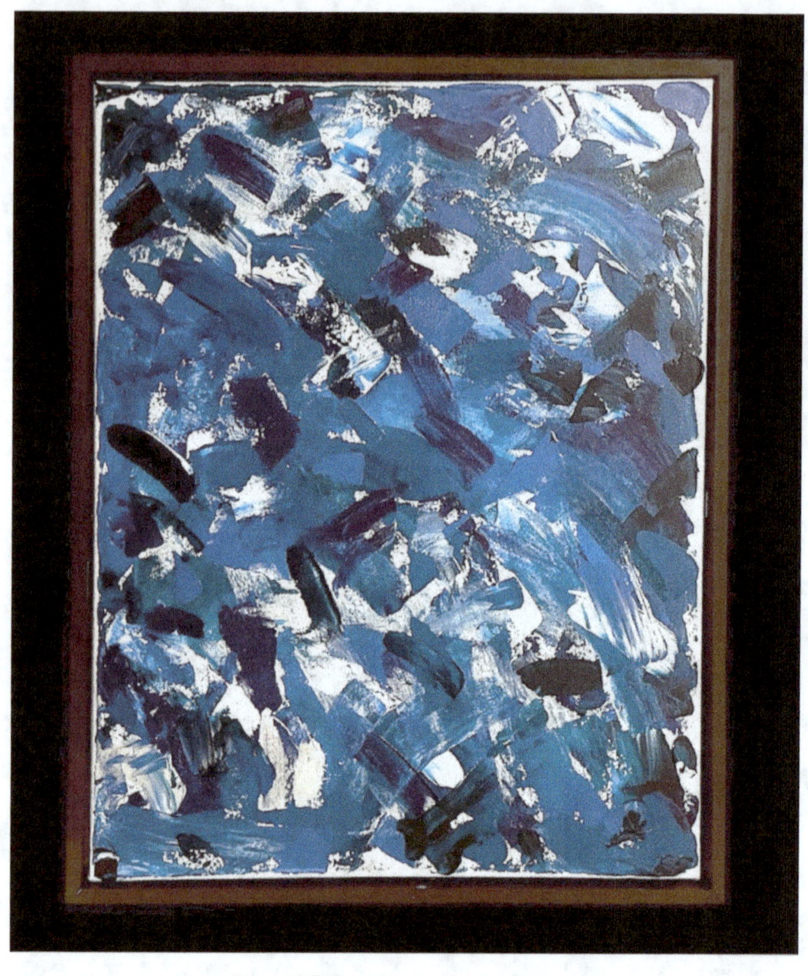

*"**Crash**", Acrylic, 16" x 20", 2022*

Tides of Grief

I told my story
Through choked sobs,
The words breaking my own heart.
The memories felt fresh on my tongue
And the tears stung of shame.
I am not yet ready to face
The torment of regret again.
I cannot run, nor hide, nor ignore
And I am unabashedly unprepared
To survive the tidal wave
roaring into shore.

I cannot breathe, I cannot wake
From this deafening nightmare
That pummels me incessantly
With insistence. Without reprieve.
I am not strong enough to withstand
The earth-shattering lightning
Searing my very soul.

All collapses.

All is still.

I watch from the eye,
the tumultuous calm.

* * *

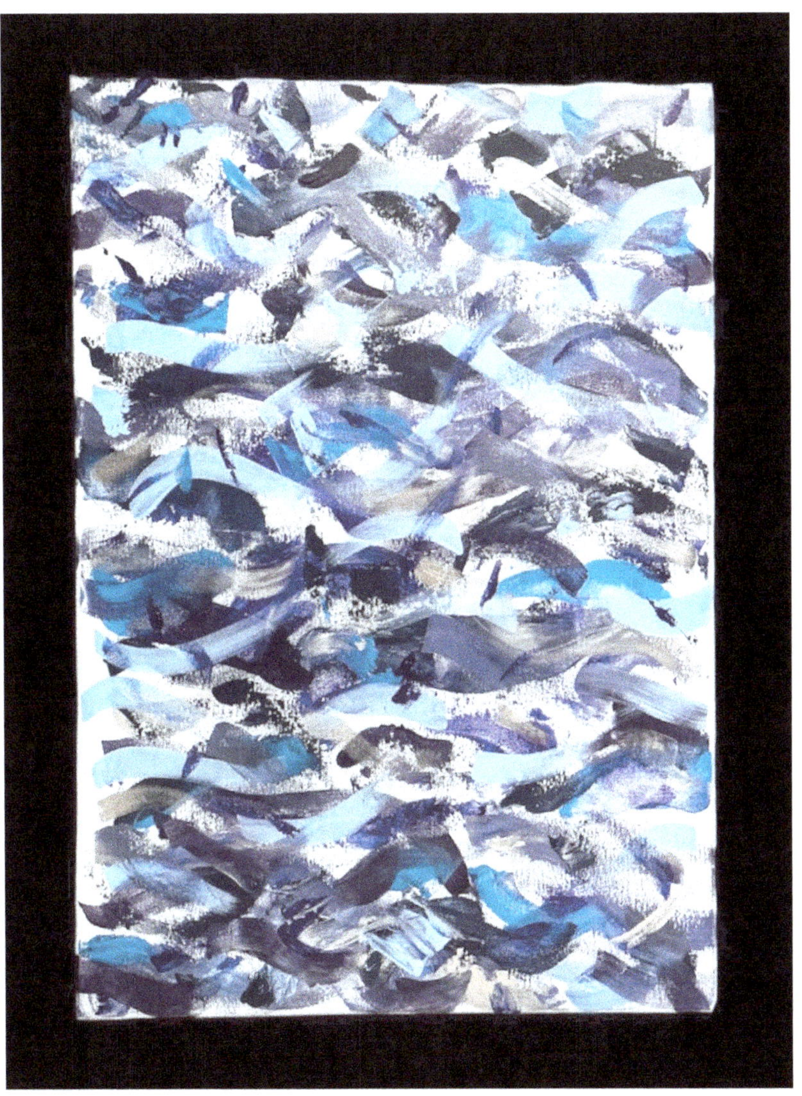

"The Breaking Wave", Acrylic, 18" x 24", 2023

Cloudy with a chance of broken

She
smiles,
but
the
sunshine
never
reaches
her
eyes.

* * *

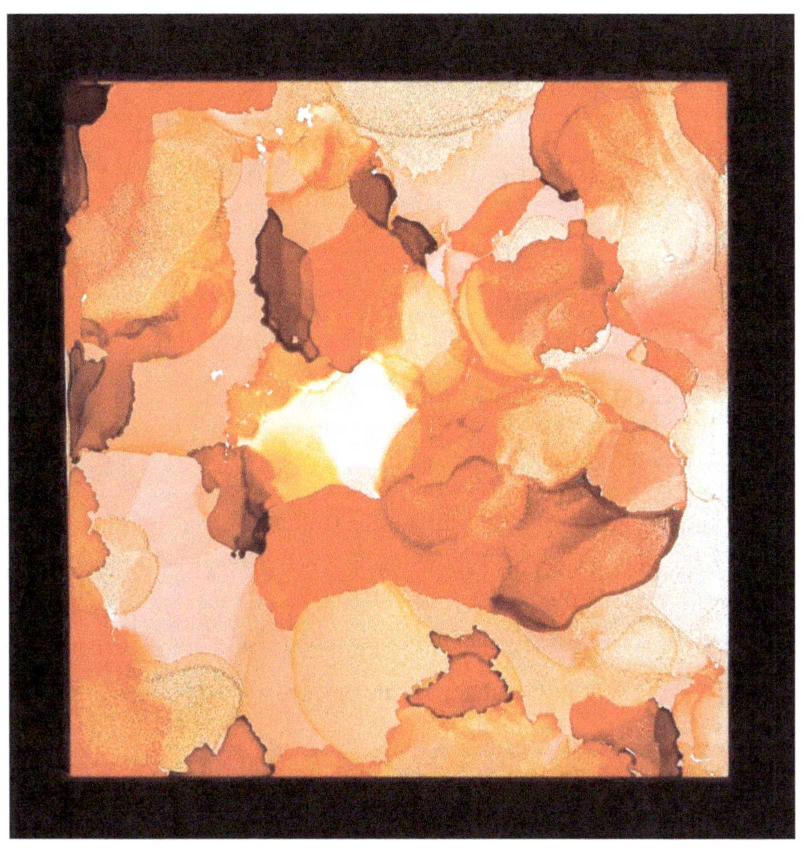

*"**Strawberry Wine**", Alcohol Inks, 6" x 6", 2021*

On Her Darkest Days

Please let me sob and let me cry
Most days I still wonder why.

Stay with me while I mourn and grieve.
It's been a lifetime without reprieve.

I'm weary and a broken mess.
But it's from all I repress.

If I'm too difficult, I will understand.
I've no other safe place to land.
But please don't leave me…
On my feet I can barely stand.

I need you on my darkest days.
I beg of you… Stay.

* * *

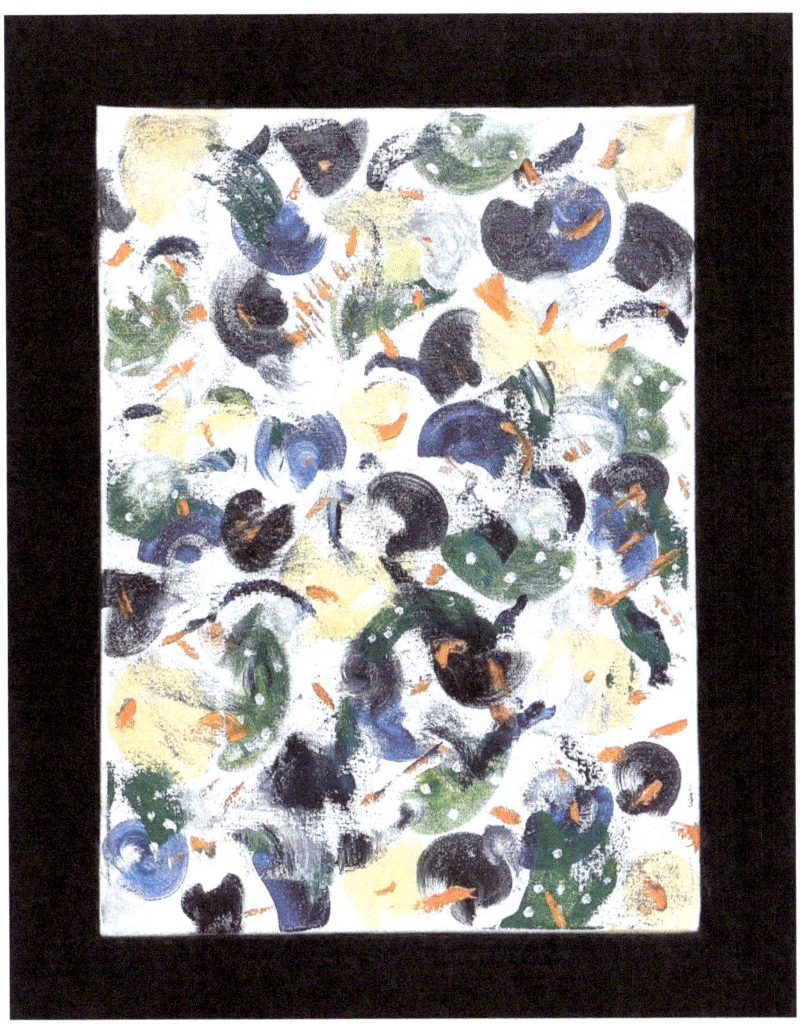

"El Caos del Paraìso", Acrylic, 12" x 16", 2023

Village of One

We constantly hear
it takes a village,
but in our culture,
the village flees
at the first signs
of grief and trauma.

Who do you turn to
when you're *too* much
for even the *bravest*?

* * *

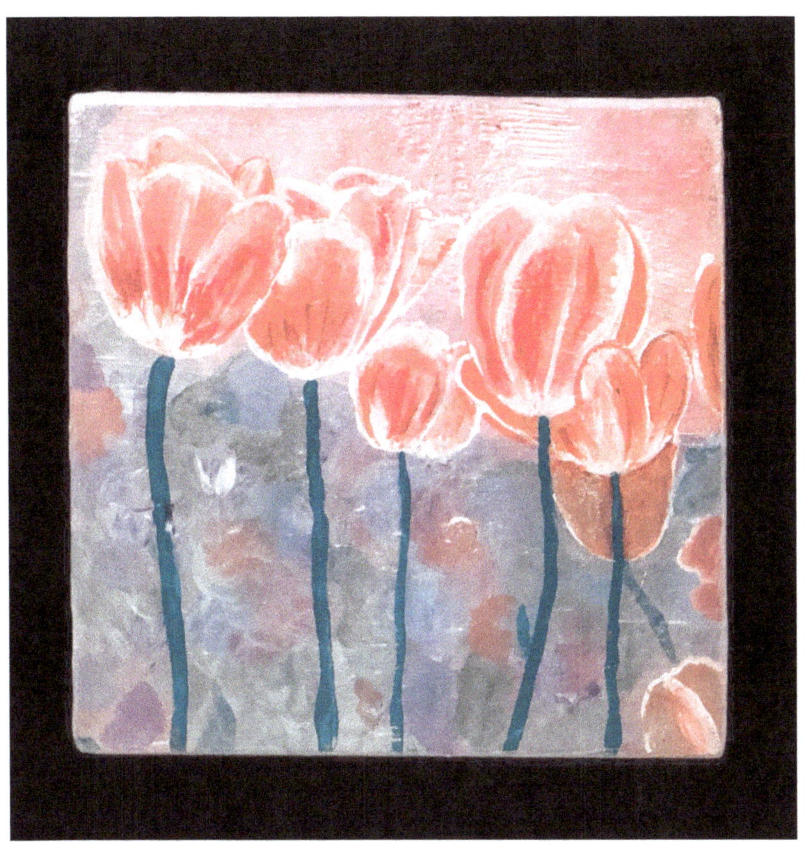

*"**Desperate for Light**", Acrylic, 3" x 3", 2020*

Chipped Paint

I loathe
my own
fragility…
the way
it chips away
in fragments
and pieces.
I am weakness
personified,
and I stretch
and break
in all my
corners
and
creases.

Gasping

I watch the world in austere silence,
held captive by this broken shell of myself.
Oh, if only I could speak the words
these mute lips hide.
Perhaps then, I could breathe again.

* * *

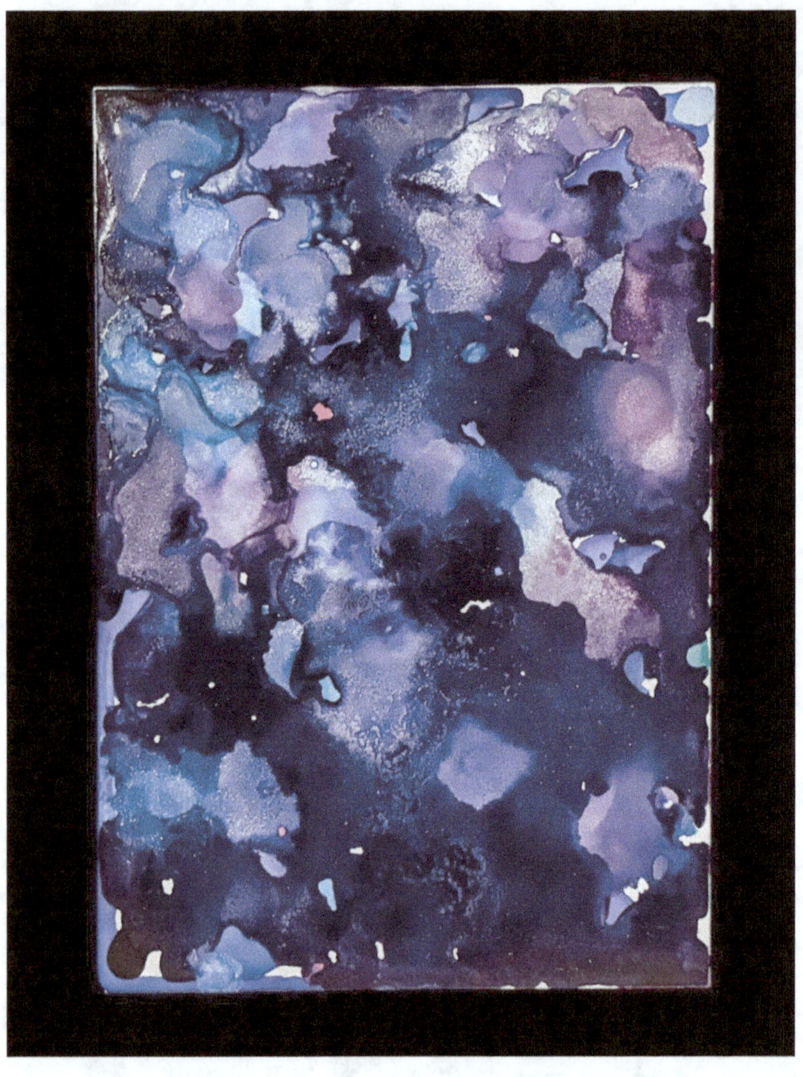

*"**Deeper**", Alcohol Inks, 5" x 7", 2022*

The Disappearing Reflection

She stared at me knowingly
Her wounded eyes took me in.
She reached her hand out
to touch my cheek
in a familiar kind of way.
The color was completely drained
from the picture of her face,
The burden of life clawed at her skin,
Leaving her battered and bruised.
And yet she whispered in a hush,
"Please don't give up on me."
She turned away in grief,
As if seeing me hurt her heart.
I called out to the broken girl…
Reaching for her hand,
But she simply faded away…
Because the wounded girl is me.

* * *

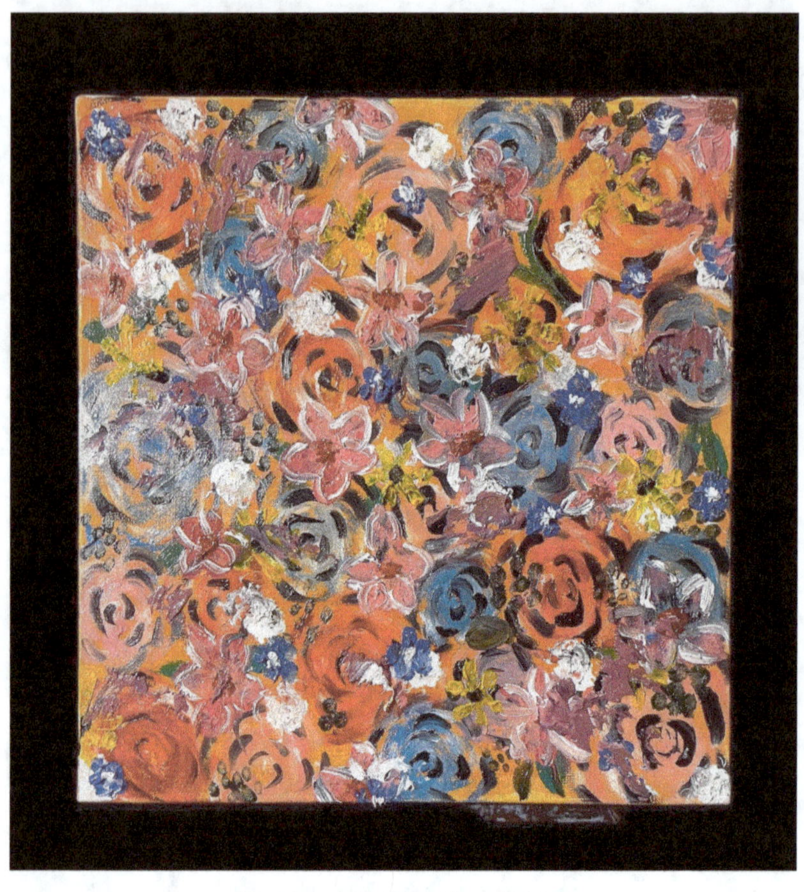

"Potpourri", Oils, 8" x 8", 2023

Flash!

I took a million pictures of you
Trying to capture your new face
But I look at those pictures now in shock.
I don't remember them, not a trace…

* * *

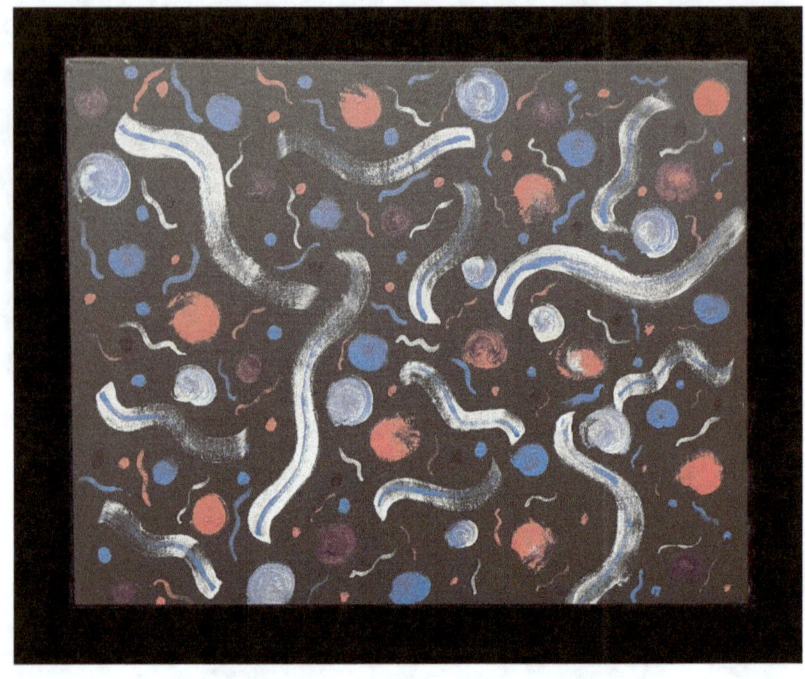

"Hello and Goodbye", Acrylic, 16" x 20", 2022

See Me

The hush of solitude lingers again.
A grateful yet unwelcome silence.
I can feel my senses heightened
As my chest constricts with quiet sobs.

This deafening loneliness
wraps its arms around me
And I cannot see the light anymore.

All is dark.
I beckon a hint of flame,
But alas, the flicker dies
Taking the remaining joy with it.

I need to breathe,
But it comes in distressed gasps.
I grasp for someone's hand to help,
But this is my burden to bear.

So alone I remain
In this dark, suffocating cocoon.
I am bound by my own battle wounds

Invisible to all inquiring eyes.

I beg of you, please,
bear witness to me,
though I'm tattered
by the years of internal war.

You don't have to save me.
Just please…see me as I am.

* * *

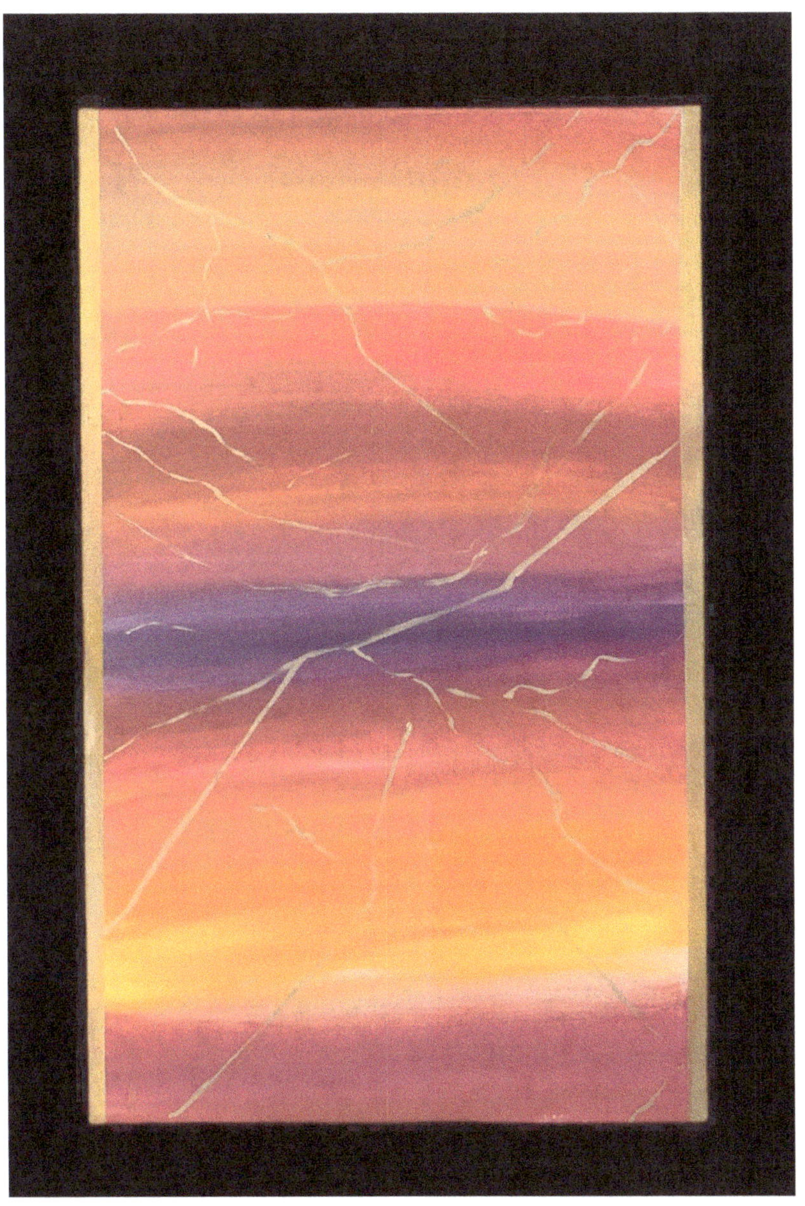

*"**Keep Your Eyes to the Sky**", Acrylic, 24" x 36", 2022, finished 2023*

Synonyms

I could use a
thousand different words
to tell you how sad I am.
But that would over complicate it.

I am sad.
I'm sad in my bones.
In my heart.
In my flesh and blood.

I am sad in a way that swallows me whole.
I'm so sad, I might never be okay.
I'm sad, and I can't run from it.

I am not morose.
I am not devastated.
I am not sorrowful.

I'm just really sad, okay?

* * *

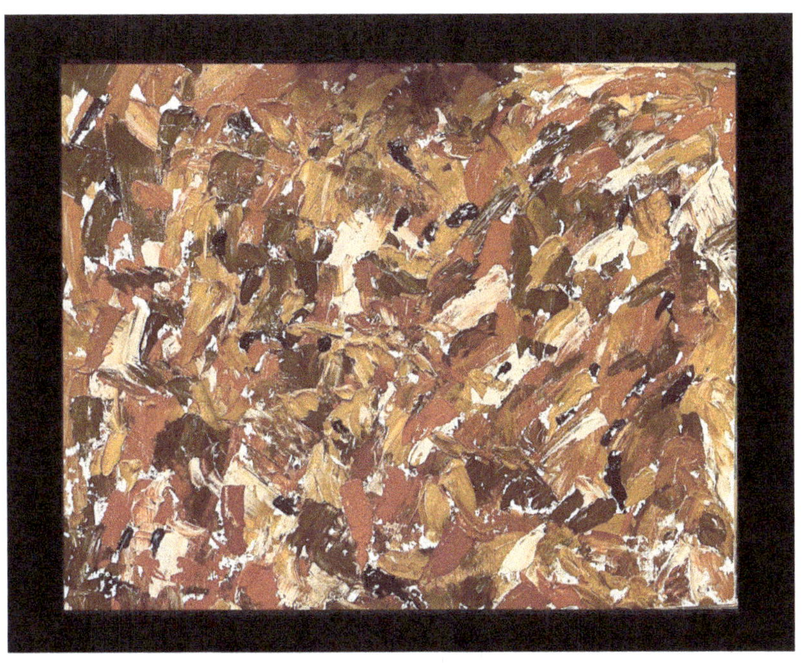

"Everything is Fine", Acrylic, 16" x 20", 2022

The Weight Of It All

I never knew
that you could
simultaneously feel
so empty
yet astonishingly
H E A V Y
at the same time.

* * *

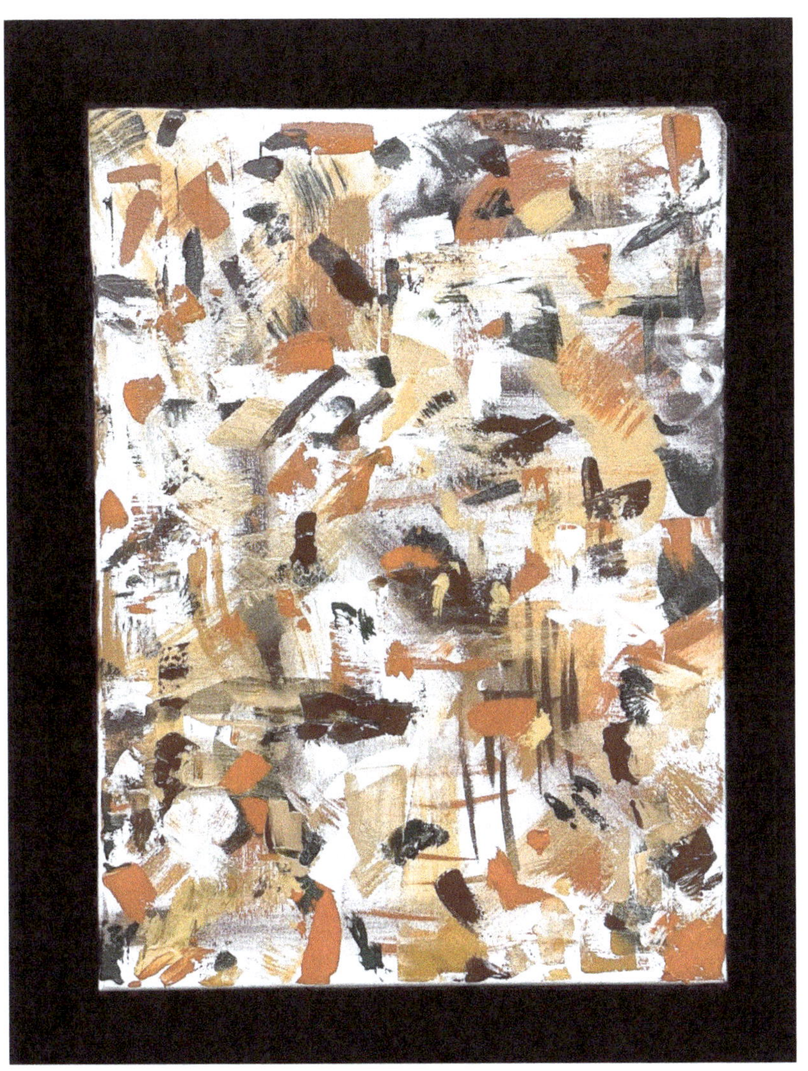

*"**Lost and Found**", Acrylic, 18" x 24, 2023*

Gone Away

Suddenly, the anger is more than I can bear.
I am drowning in it, I can barely gasp for air.

I've picked up the pieces that fell to the ground,
While there was nobody else around.

I've built myself up, a column strong,
And everyone forgot what was wrong.

It's not their fault for living their lives,
They're busy being mothers and wives.

But they left me so very alone,
While I suffered in isolation at home.

Rendered unable to function from trauma,
They only saw the smiling mama.

I breathe and remember, it wasn't their fault.
Guess it's time for me to be my own adult.

But my inner child screams, "Please just hold me."

That young part, the little girl, about age three.

She's scared, and hurt, and she doesn't understand.
Was this all part of the plan?

She cries again and vows to survive.
After all, maybe only the baby needs to *thrive*.

* * *

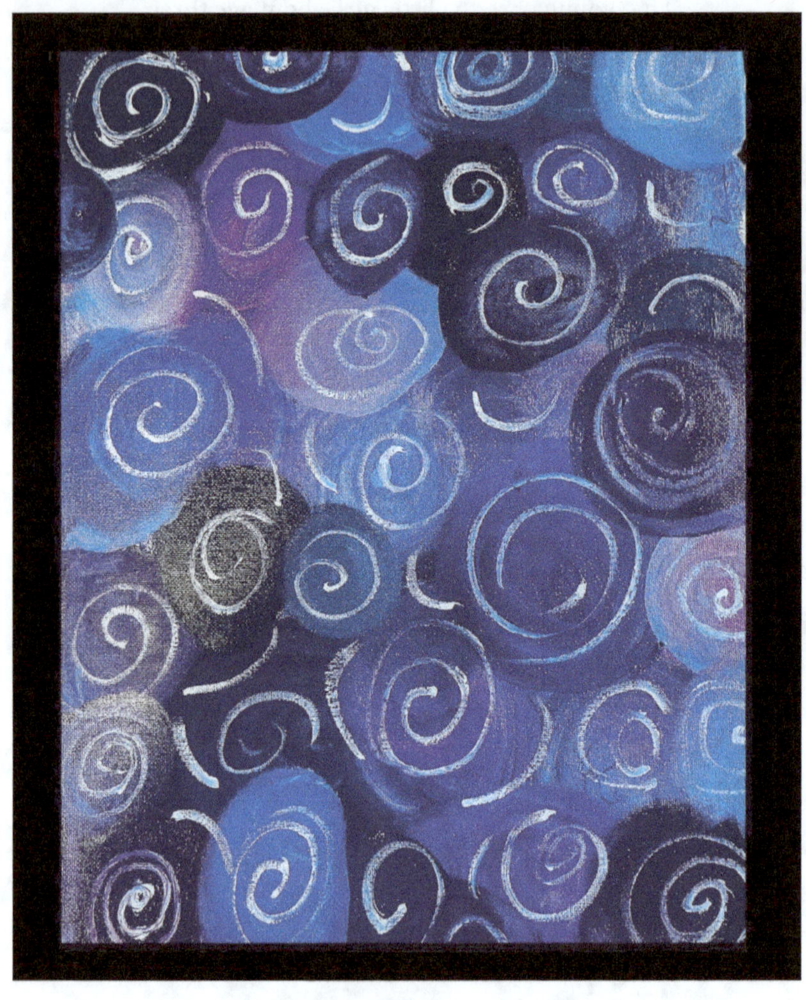

"Swirling Mind", Acrylic, 2022

Well Meaning

"Enjoy every minute."
That phrase became my kryptonite.
Because the truth was I hated a lot of it.

For the first nine months,
I was traumatized, and drowning,
But any time I said that to anyone,
They told me to hold onto those memories
Because they go so fast.

But I was dying inside,
And nobody told me
it was okay to not love it all.

That yes, it's rewarding,
But it's also *hard*,
And without support,
It can feel *impossible*.

I did **not** enjoy every minute.

I love my babies immensely.

And I believe them to be my most precious gifts.
But I'll be damned if I tell anyone
That postpartum was happy for me.

* * *

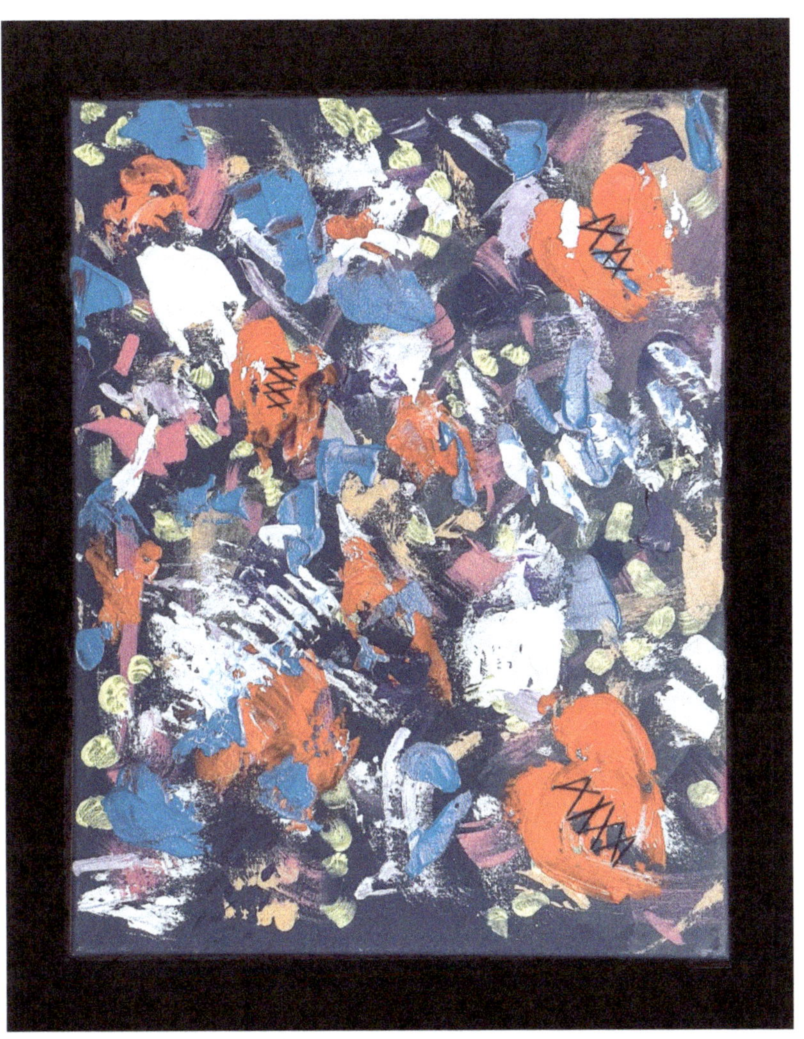

*"**Broken and Sewn**", Mixed Media, 16" x 20", 2023*

Water Her

Be gentle.
I may look
The same from afar,
But I'm different inside.
Part of me died
And I don't know
To bring her back to life.

* * *

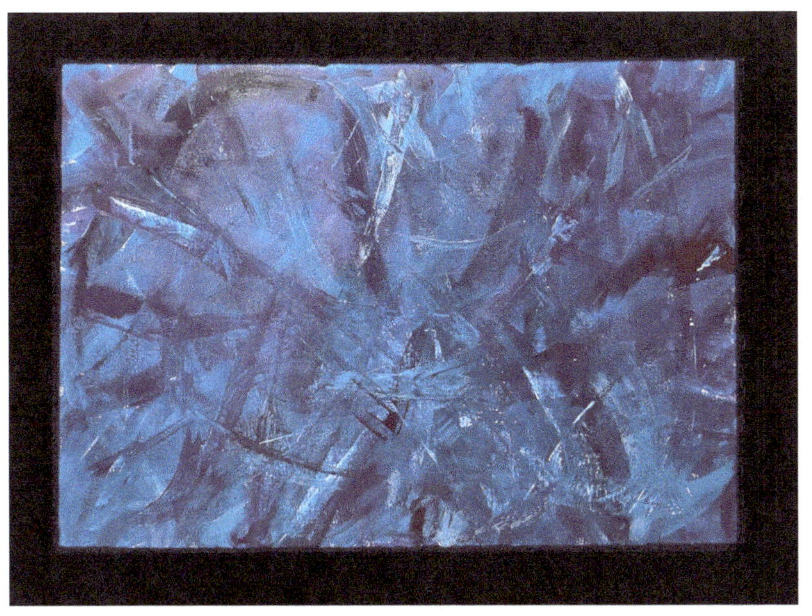

*"**In My Blue Phase**", Acrylic, 36" x 24", 2022*

Schism of Sorrow

Like a canyon,
there is a painful schism between

who I once *was*

and who I am *now*,

and no amount of hope
will repair the unbearable break.

For the valleys reach lower into the depths,
and I'm too tired to climb out again.

They say seeing the canyon
takes your breath away.

I'm still waiting to find air.

* * *

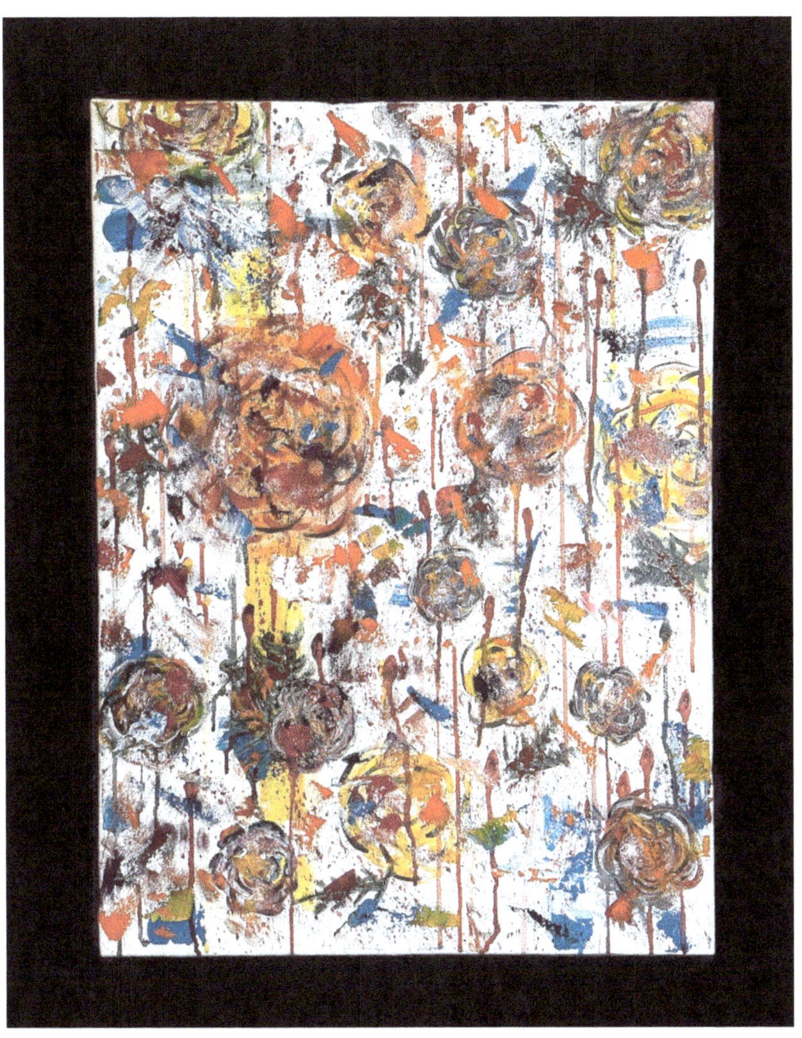

"Even the Flowers Bleed", Oils, 18" x 24", 2023

The Fantasy of Death

A chaotic, turbulent mind
leaves my heart barely clinging to life, blind.

My eyes cannot wake from this unrelenting nightmare.
My soul believes not a person out there cares.

I am trapped in my own body, ragged and weary,
My eyesight blurred, forever bleary.

The dark storm rages violently in my heart,
Angry and seething at all the ways I fall apart.

I am void of happiness, stripped of hope,
Clinging fervently to my frayed, thin rope.

I cannot hold on to this life any longer,
I cannot be what you want, I wish I was stronger.

My grasp slips, and I finally let go.
Sweet release, I fall below.

Deep in the waters, away from the sky

I fall…
I fall…
I fall…
Until in darkness I quietly lie.

Peace flows over me, the stillness surrounds,
One last breath…

the exhale profound.

* * *

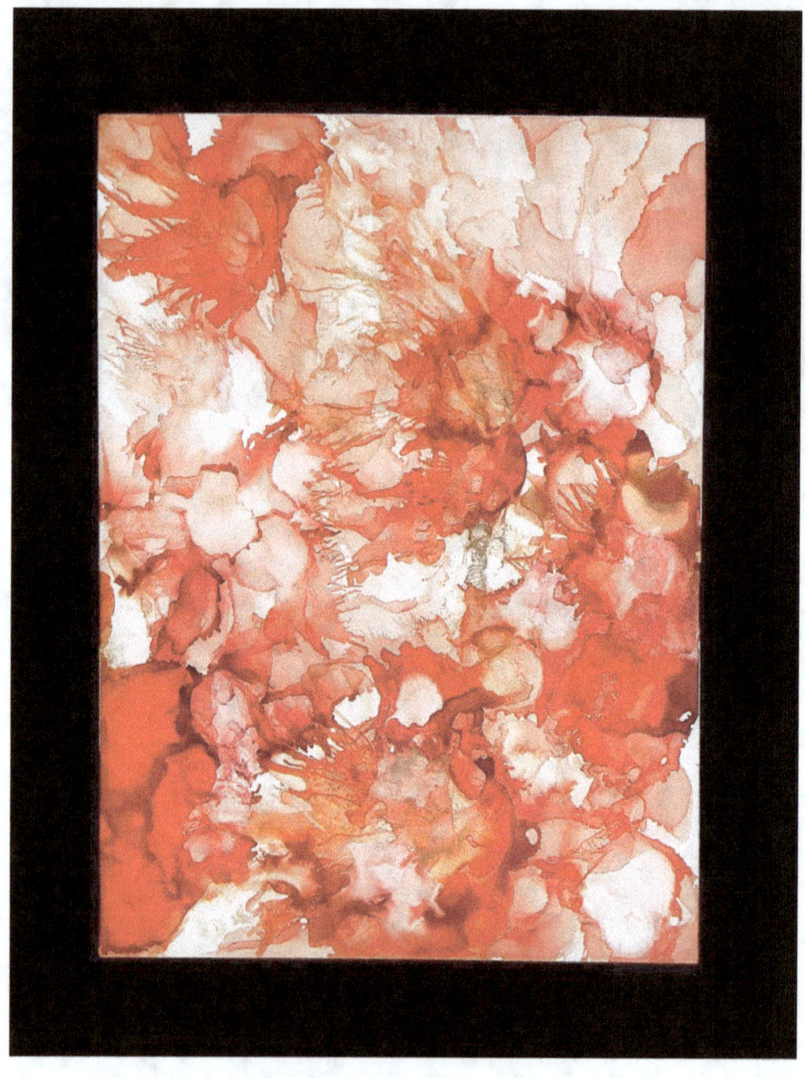

*"**Burst**", Alcohol Inks, 2022*

I Give In

She found it too painful
to exist in her own mind.
So she ran away again and again,
but the agony chased her
until it was too hard to keep going.
An excruciating surrender.

* * *

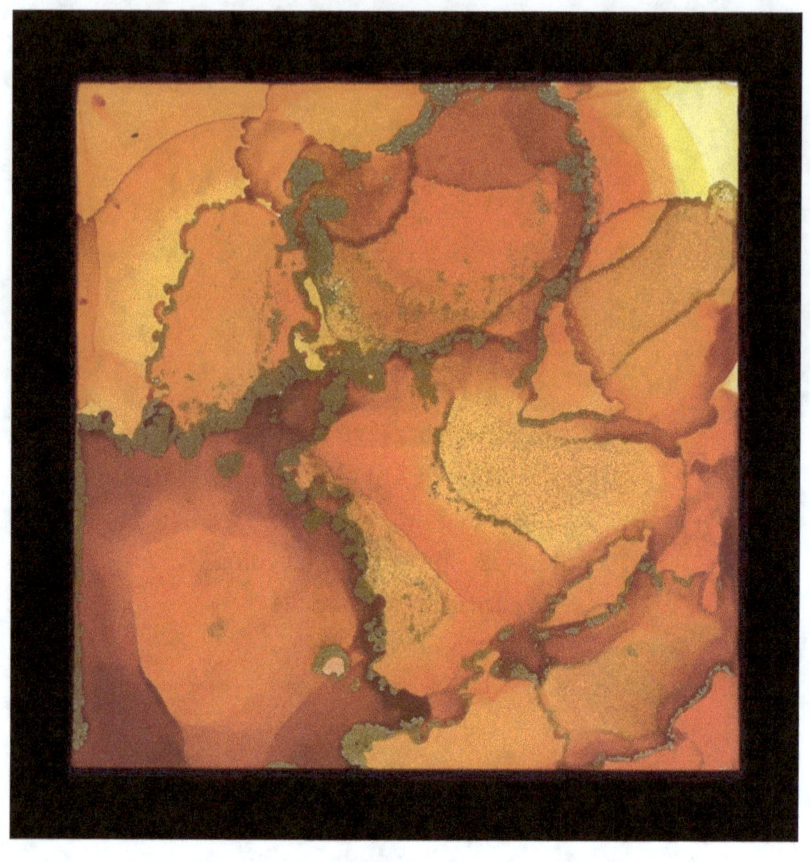

"You Are My Sunshine", Alcohol Inks, 4" x 4", 2019

Living On Scraps

My brain lives among the huddled masses of emotional poverty.
My mind is starving for peace and hungry for hope.
I beg for compassion and plead for the normalcy I so crave.
My mind is naked and shivering from neglect.
What I wouldn't give for a place to rest my weary mind.
But that which I crave is just out of reach.
Scared and alone, I crumple beneath the weight of this wearisome
state of mind.
My brain screams, "Please help me!" but nobody comes.
I am condemned to this life, and there is no escape.

* * *

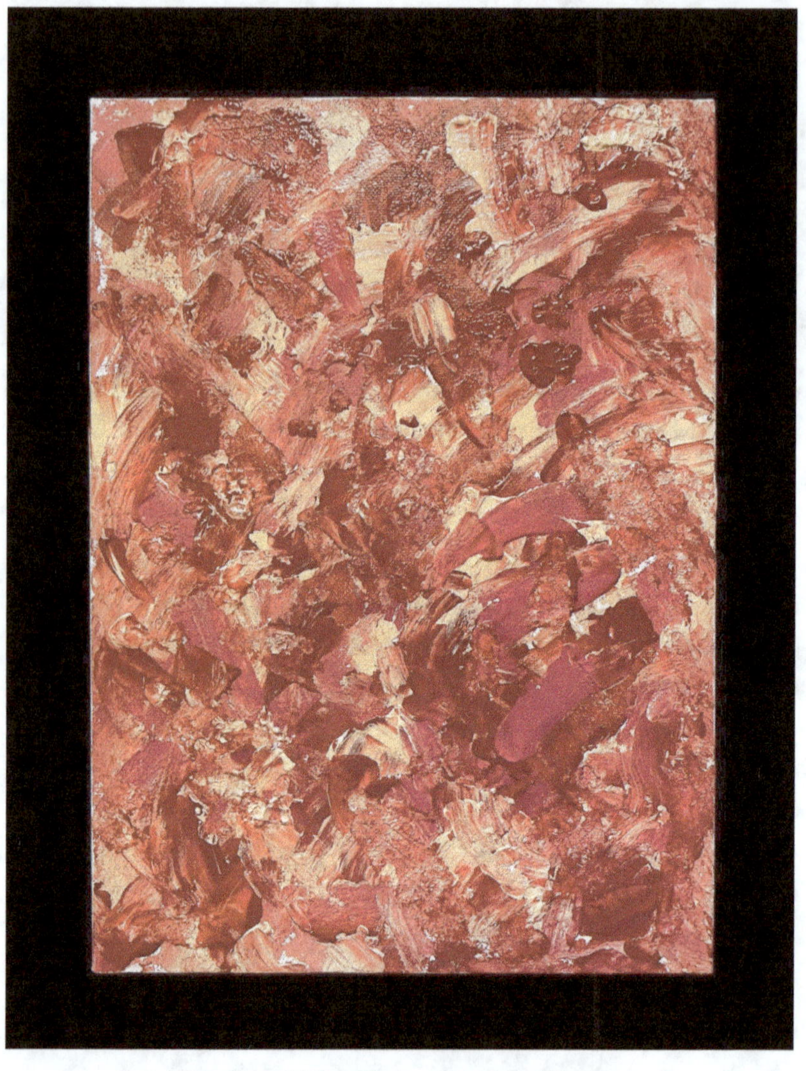

"Flesh and Blood", Acrylic, 9" x 12", 2022

Who Was She?

I'd
give
anything
to
know
the
girl
I
was
before
I
B
R
O
K
E...

***

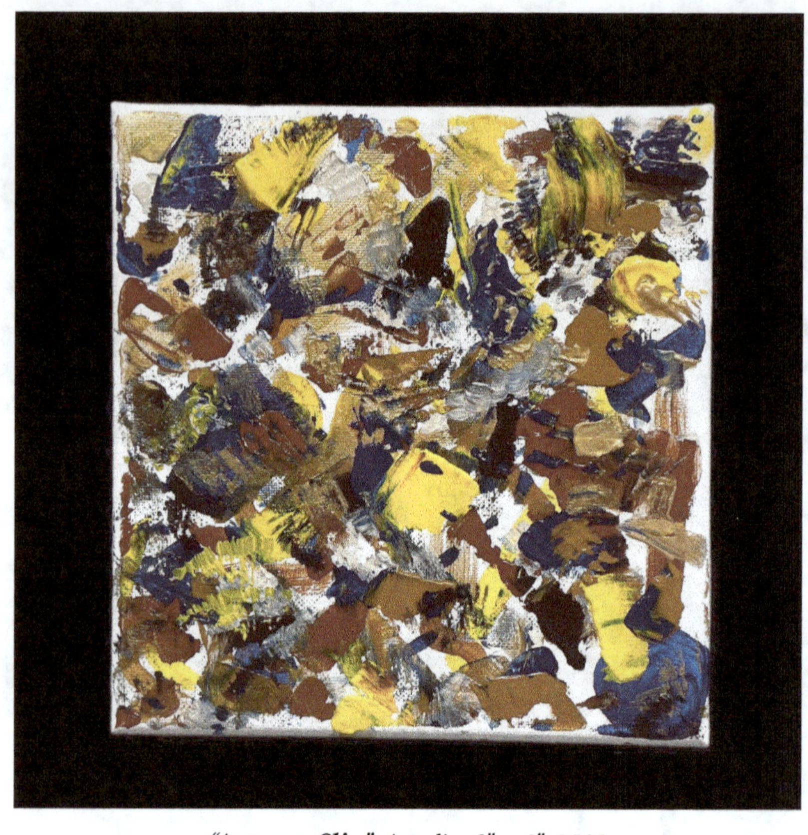

*"**Autumn Slip**", Acrylic, 8" x 8", 2023*

A Mom, Forgot

She said, I swear I'm fine.
And that was a pretty good line.

But that truth only lasted a while,
Before you could see her fading smile.

And to the camera, she'd smile and wave,
But her cheeks were gaunt and began to cave.

She didn't eat, she didn't sleep,
She just fed the baby on *repeat*.

She hugged her knees and prayed to God…
But God only gave her a nod.

And so her silent tears became her song,
Of everything about motherhood that was wrong.

Because there should be joy when a baby happens,
But nothing was happy once it was all in action.

The baby cried endlessly for hours,

And I swear… that cry, her soul, it devoured.

She longed for someone to hold her tight.
To tell her not to give up the fight.

But she was invisible to everyone she knew,
Because, "Look at the adorable baby in blue!"

You hugged the baby and squealed with joy,
But what the hell was this ploy?

I didn't expect it. I didn't prepare!
God, it doesn't seem fair!

I'm not cut out for this, I'm a shit mom.
It was supposed to be wonderful, but it exploded like a bomb.

And the husband I thought I knew so well,
Became part of my invisible hell.

So the baby cried, and I cried, too.
Because, what's it to you?

You don't care whether I'm here or not.
I'm simply a mom, forgot.

* * *

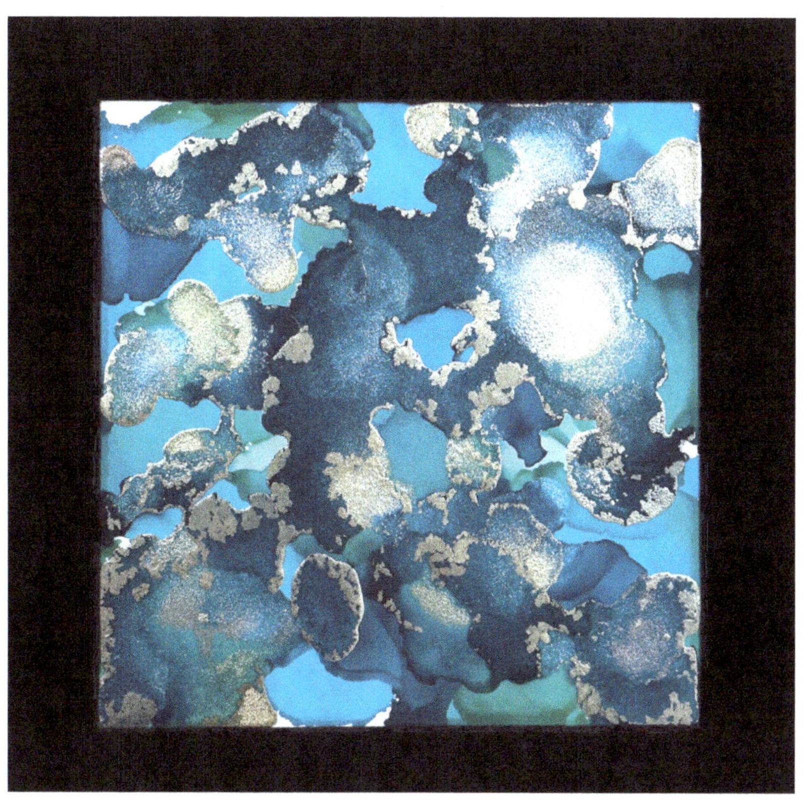

"Emerald City", Alcohol Inks, 4" x 4", 2023

V

Love, Marriage, A Baby in a Carriage…Then What?

Zap!

We tried the whole first week to put him down,
So we could simply move around
To just hold hands, to hug to kiss,
But we always missed.

His cry would start,
We'd leap apart,
And because baby comes first,
The shock of the separation is the worst.

* * *

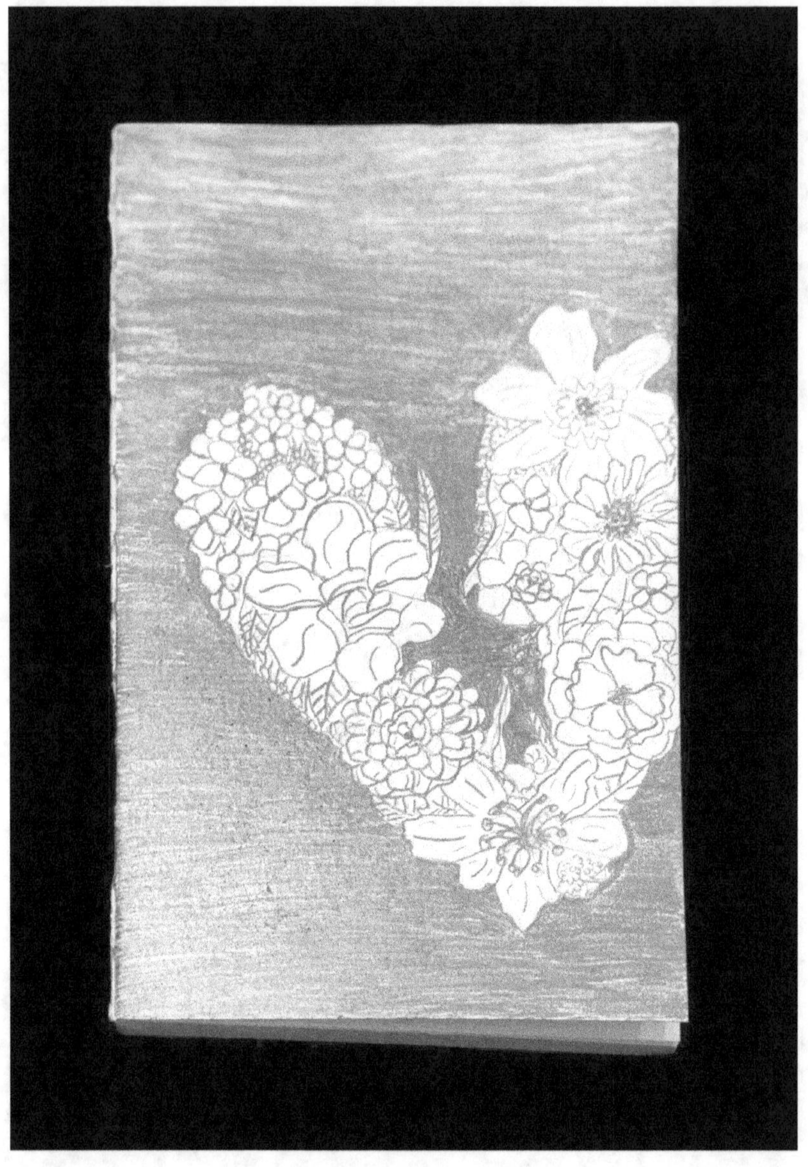

*"**Split**", Graphite, 2024*

Who Put Me in Charge?

You left me alone with this tiny creature,
And I don't know them, where is the teacher?

I'm not yet healed, I can't seem to stop bawling,
I was just sewn closed, I'm barely crawling.

Why did you leave when I needed you the most?
Of myself, I'm just a ghost.

Please come back, please take care of me,
I'm not surviving, can't you see?

I beg of you, help me find my way,
Everything in the world looks gray.

You left me alone, you left me sad,
Why aren't you being a dad?

* * *

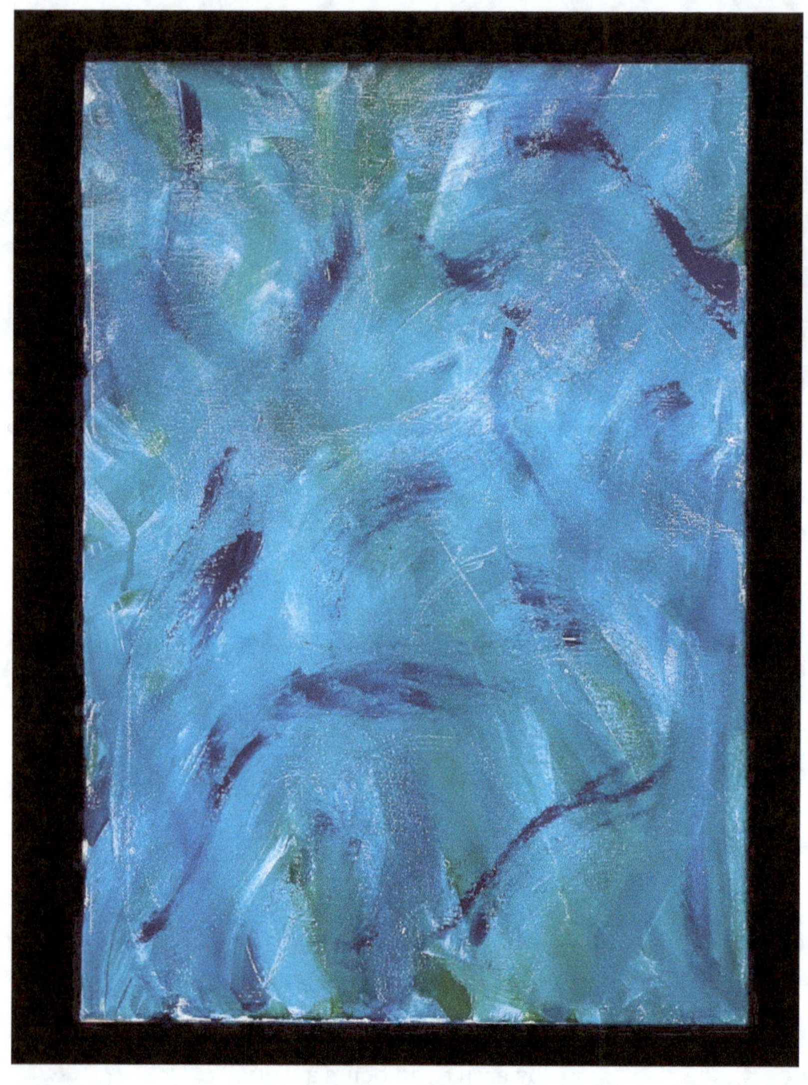

"Twisted Mist", Oils, 12" x 16", 2023

I Dare You

She cried for me,
Screaming for her mama,
We had both just been through
So much trauma.

Grasping her tight,
He clutched her in his arms,
I reached for her,
My brain, all alarms.

"Please let me hold her,
She needs me right now."
But to let me touch her,
He wouldn't allow.

I pleaded for her presence
As her screams grew,
I needed to soothe her,
I knew what to do.

But he shoved me away,
His hands pushed me hard,

Like he was somehow
Her rightful bodyguard.

"I've got it," he growled
And kept me at a distance,
While I sobbed and sobbed,
Begging with insistence.

I panicked, and yelled,
"Give me my fucking baby!"
And he looked at me in disgust,
Like I wasn't a damn lady.

He handed her
to me with force,
And scoffed in my face
It was always my fault, of course.

I held her shrieking body,
I sobbed and sobbed,
In that moment everything changed,
Our safety had been robbed.

* * *

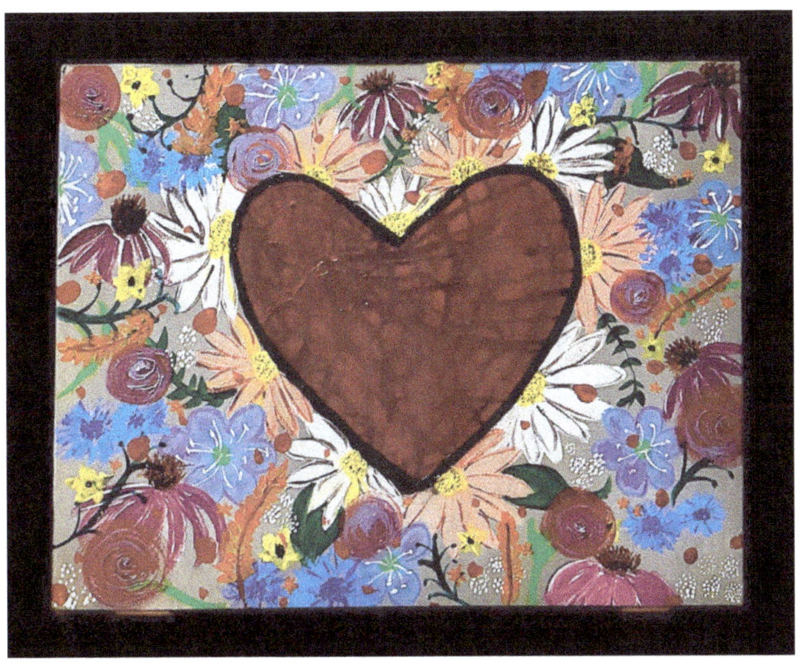

*"**Laid to Rest**", Acrylic, 12" x 16", 2024*

A Different Wife

Who is that in the mirror?
She's not the wife I knew,
Who would want her anymore?
Every part of her grew.

I can't be seen,
I'll die of shame…
If my husband sees me,
Naked and plain.

My scar is tender,
My tummy sags,
The only things that fit me
Are the spit up rags.

Please don't push me to do this.
The trauma is making it feel like a threat.
I know you miss me,
But please…I'm not ready yet.

* * *

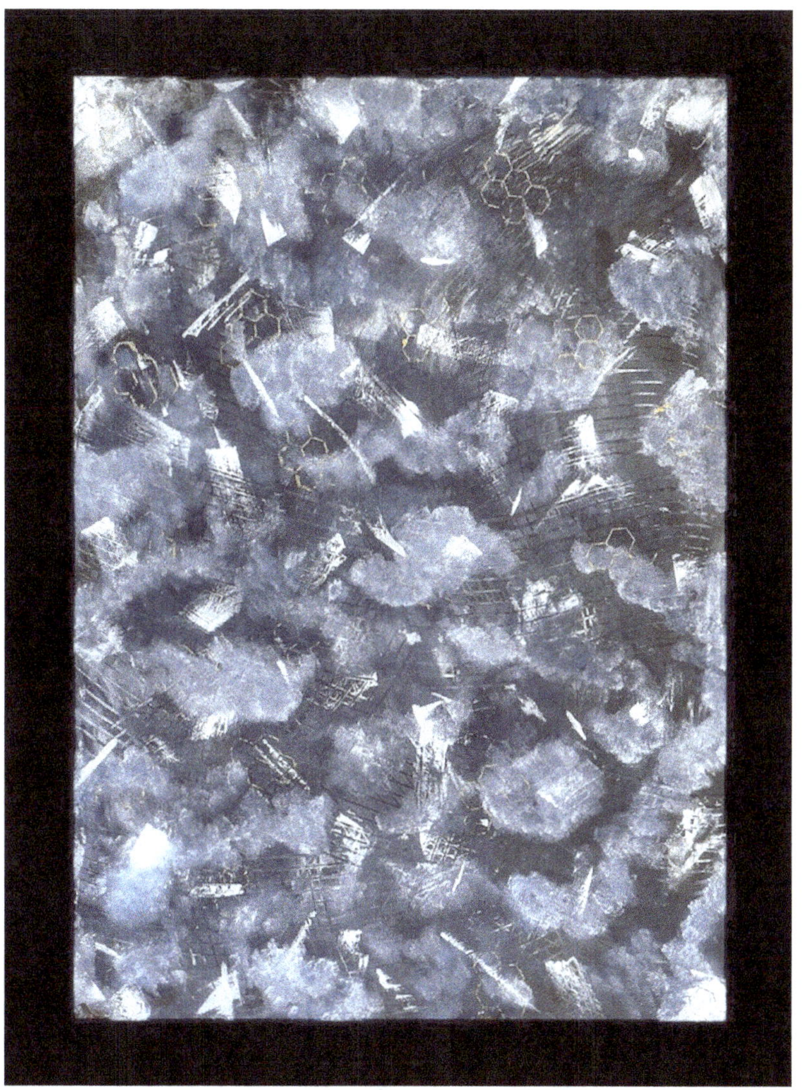

"The Tempest of Reckoning", Acrylic, 36" x 48", 2023

Favors Due

Sex is only just for you,
It's all about what I owe, what's due.
It isn't what's good for me,
It's no longer about my needs.

You have expectations,
You extend invitations,
But I don't want you to try,
Please, I almost just died.

What if I get pregnant again?
What would I do, what then?
You want another baby, I know,
But I was just open and sewn.

Please don't push,
I can't do this in a rush,
I'm not ready for you,
I'm sorry…I thought you knew.

* * *

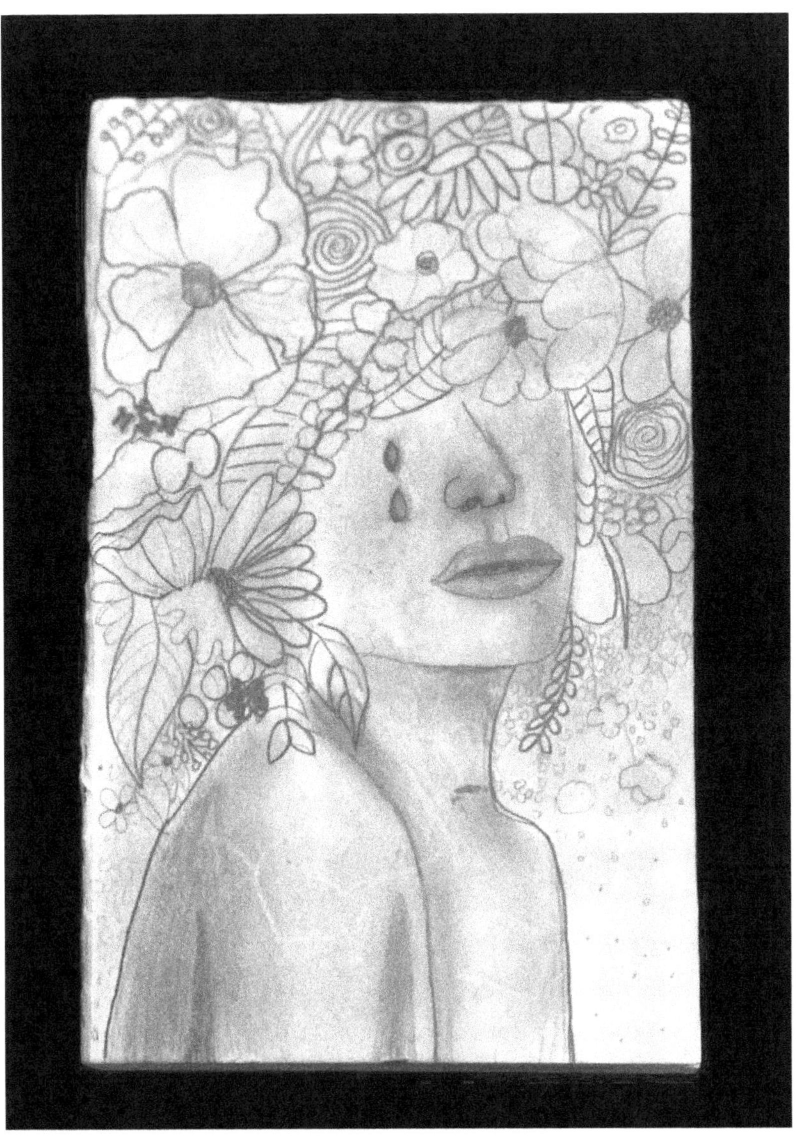

"In There Somewhere", Graphite, 2024

The Worst Betrayal

You left me when I needed you the most,
And you didn't think twice,
About how it would be for me,
While you went back to your life.

I cried so many tears,
Because I needed you there,
But you had work to do,
You didn't care.

I hoped you'd see me
Crying on the floor,
And realize I wasn't okay,
Like I was before.

But you put your head
In the clouds in the sky,
Drowning me and the baby out,
So YOU could get by.

I thought it was my fault,
I thought I did something wrong,

THE WORST BETRAYAL

But really, you didn't know how to help,
So you merely meandered along.

I resent you for that,
I hate that you were gone,
But the baby needs me now,
It's almost dawn.

* * *

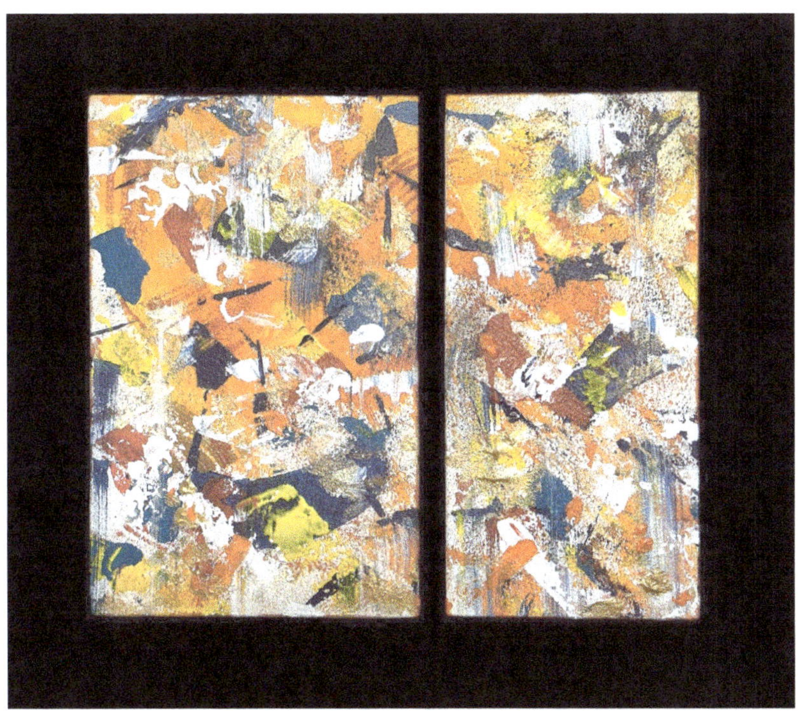

"Two Can't Tango", *Acrylic, 2023*

Rich Resentment

I hated you a little bit,
That you didn't have to go through it,
That you could move on,
Because, "It all turned out okay,
Time to move forward."
But I couldn't move at all.
And that's where we broke.
I stayed behind,
And you didn't care.

* * *

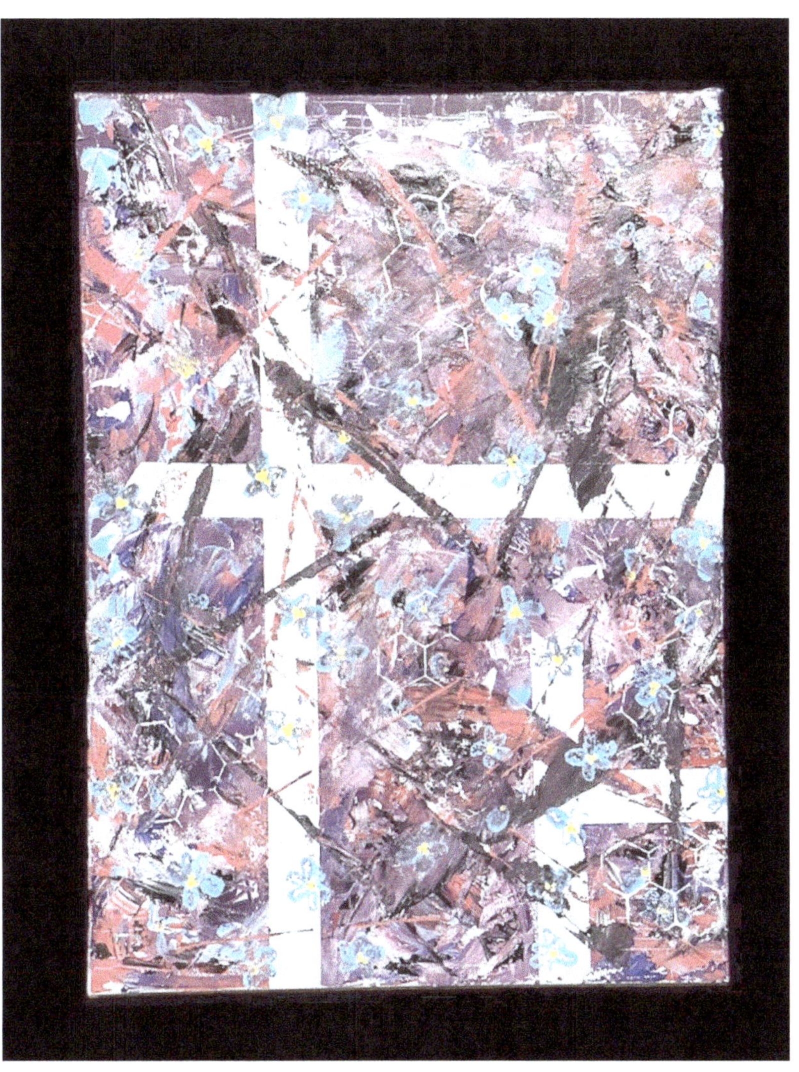

"In the Wake of the Tempest", Acrylic, 18" x 24", 2023

I Choose Me and Us Three

I made a choice to leave that day,
For many years he had paved the way.

I didn't notice when we began,
How hot and dysregulated his temper ran.

I guess I always believed,
He was as good as I perceived.

But he was always masking it well,
And it suddenly dissolved to hell.

I shame myself for not seeing the signs,
I believed our values to be aligned.

He became a man I didn't know,
And his words became blow after blow.

I left because I could not stay,
I didn't deserve to suffer and pay.

I'm scared, I'm lost, I'm sad for my heart,

But I know deep down we're better apart.

Our kids shouldn't learn that love should be pained,
I hate the hurt, but lesson gained.

* * *

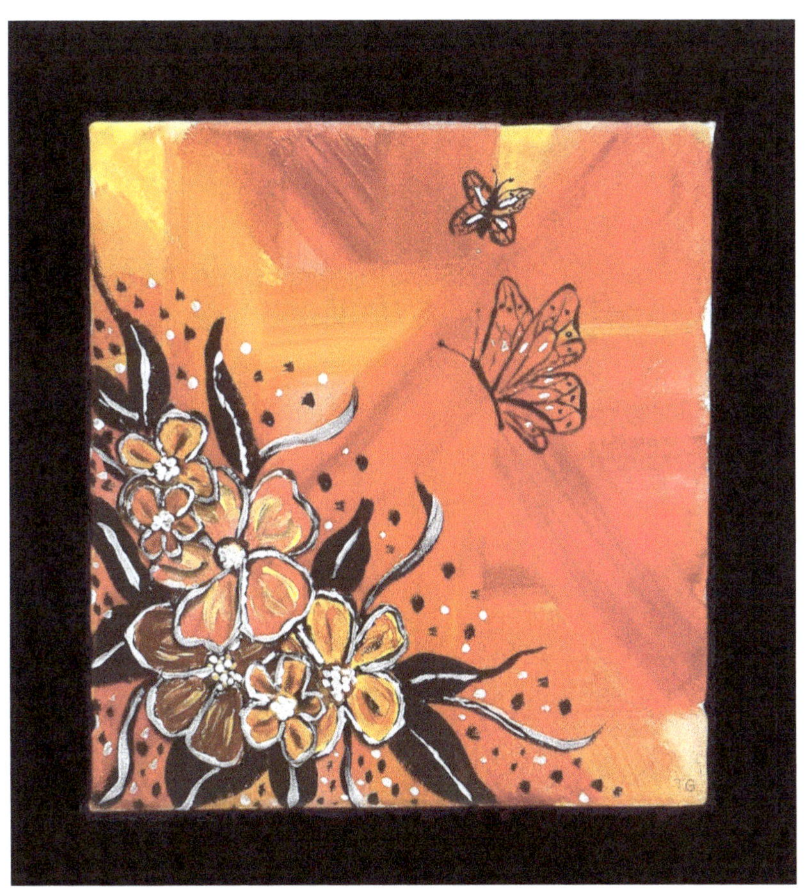

"Freedom From Fear", Mixed Media, 6" x 6", 2023

VI

Finding the Light

Rain of Relief

The sky gives itself permission to cry.
Perhaps so should I.

***

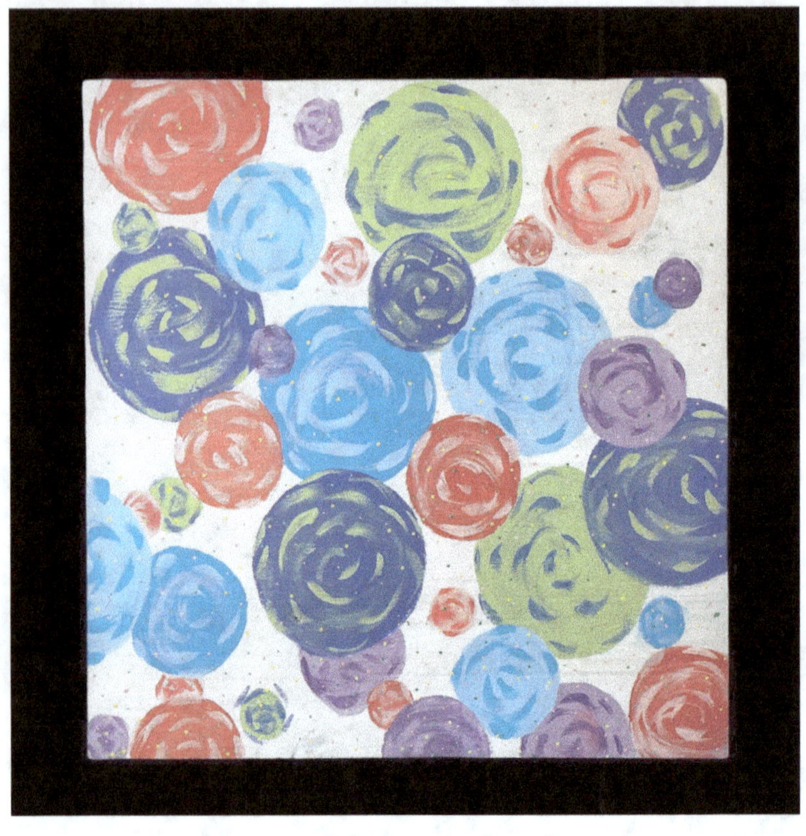

"Best Friends", Acrylic, 18" x 18", 2023

Temporary Beautiful Belly

"Look at you, you're glowing from head to toe!"
"…You haven't lost the baby weight? Oh no…"

People worship your body when your belly is full,
A joyful sight to behold.

But after the sweet baby is born,
they're more interested in the clothes you've worn.

They don't care that it took almost ten months to grow.
For some reason, they think your body, they're owed.

They say diet and exercise will make you feel whole.
And that you'll only find misery at the bottom of a bowl.

But even after birth, when I couldn't eat,
and I tried to lose weight on repeat,
nothing was ever good enough,
because they assumed my mouth I stuffed.

And if you don't lose the baby pudge,
Their ugly opinions won't budge.

My body was someone's home…
and now it's incredibly alone.

It feels barren, soft, saggy and sad.
And yet, over my pant size, you're mad.

Give me a break, I'm not here to appease,
Your assessment of my chubby knees.

It took almost a year to bring that baby here.
Please don't make me feel bad about how I appear.

I don't owe you a summer tummy.
I'm too busy being somebody's mummy.

Give it a rest after all I've been through,
Because weight is the least interesting thing about you.

* * *

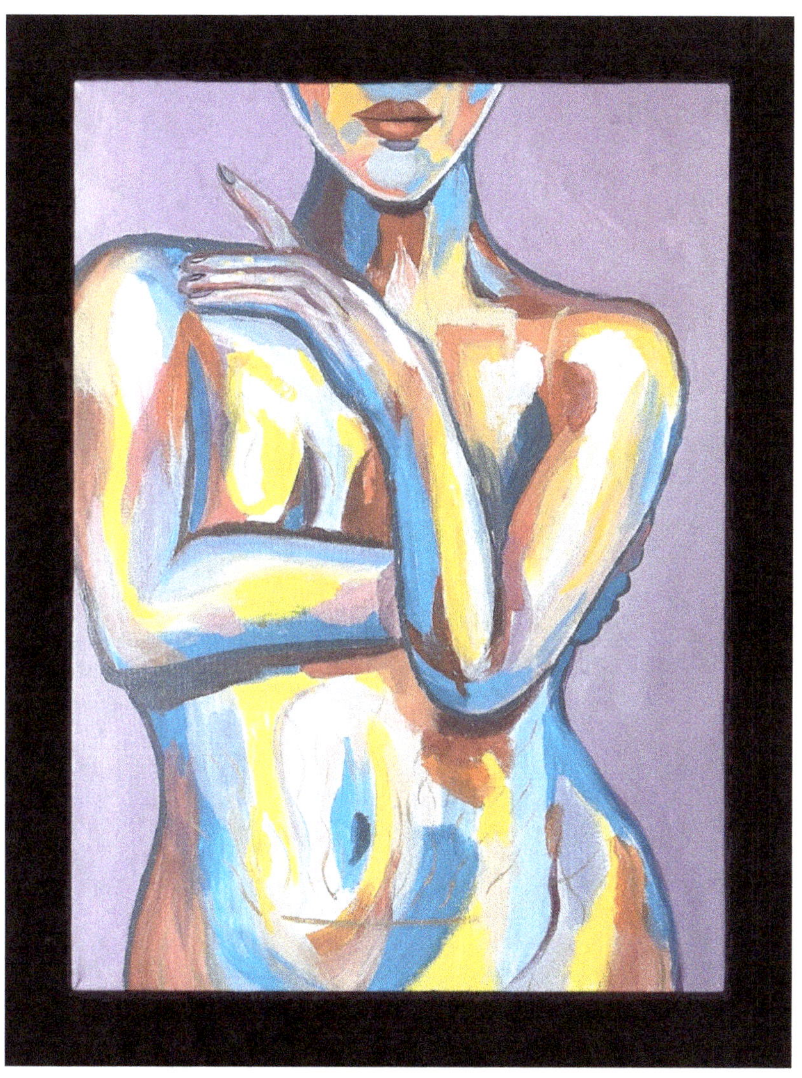

*"**Warrior Mama**", Acrylic, 16" x 20", 2023*

Wish For The Wounded

May you *inhale* the
courage you need
to *exhale* your **truth**.

* * *

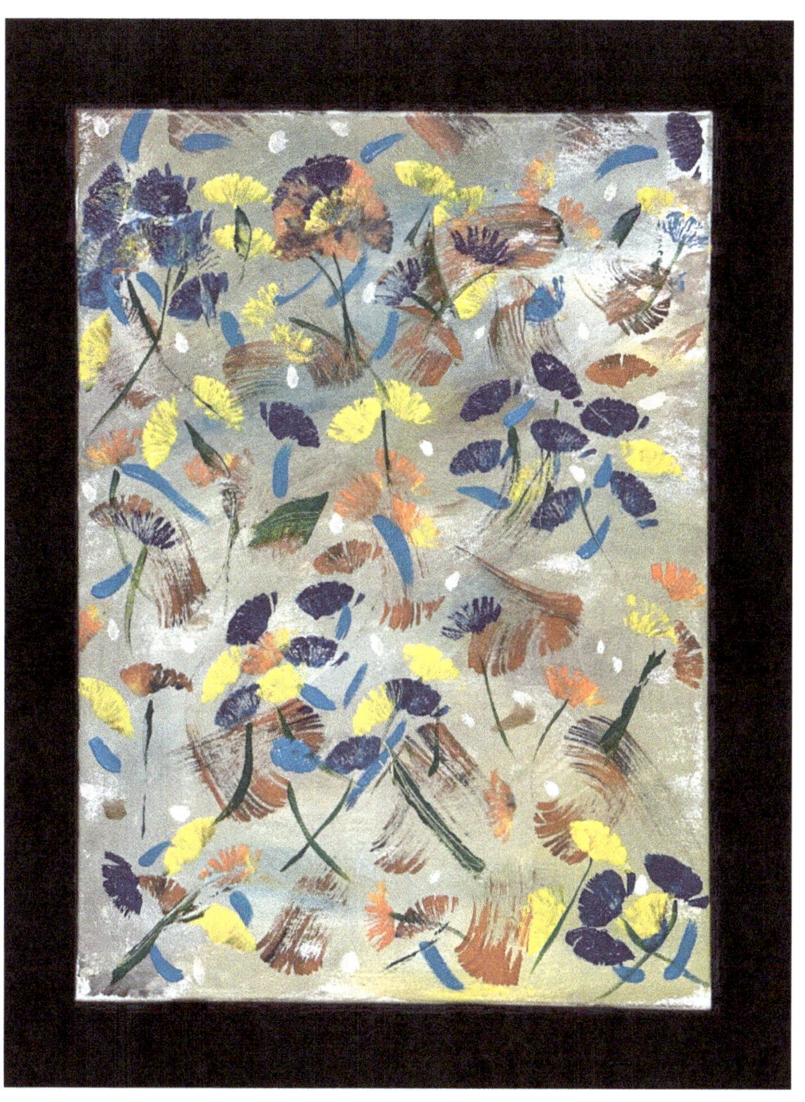

"Beneath the Hidden Flowers", Acrylic, 18" x 24", 2023

The Blessing of Art and Therapy

I painted blood,
I stood back to see
The picture of birth,
Stood there haunting me.

Brush strokes quick,
A frenzied pace,
While thick hot tears
Ran down my face.

My brush fell away
Clattering to the ground,
I panicked breathlessly
Without a sound.

I saw my grief,
My trauma, too,
In all the specific details
I just drew.

I wanted to scream
And rip at my shirt,

Finally realizing
Just how much it hurt.

And I turned to her,
Just witnessing me,
Acknowledging a strength
I could not yet see.

I was broken, bruised,
And scared to the bone.
But with my grief,
I was no longer alone.

* * *

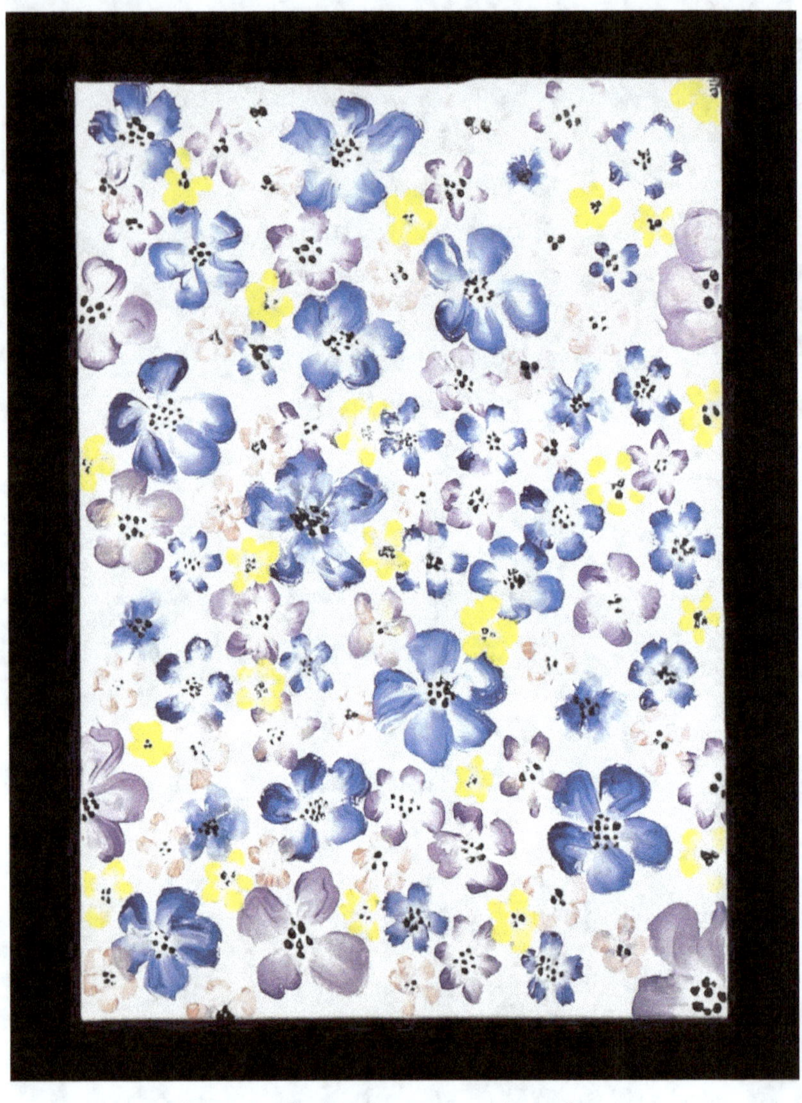

*"**Let Me Blossom**", Acrylic, 18" x 24", 2023*

What If?

What if
I stopped
racing myself
to an imaginary
finish line
of recovery,
and instead
allowed myself
the time
I need
to grieve?

* * *

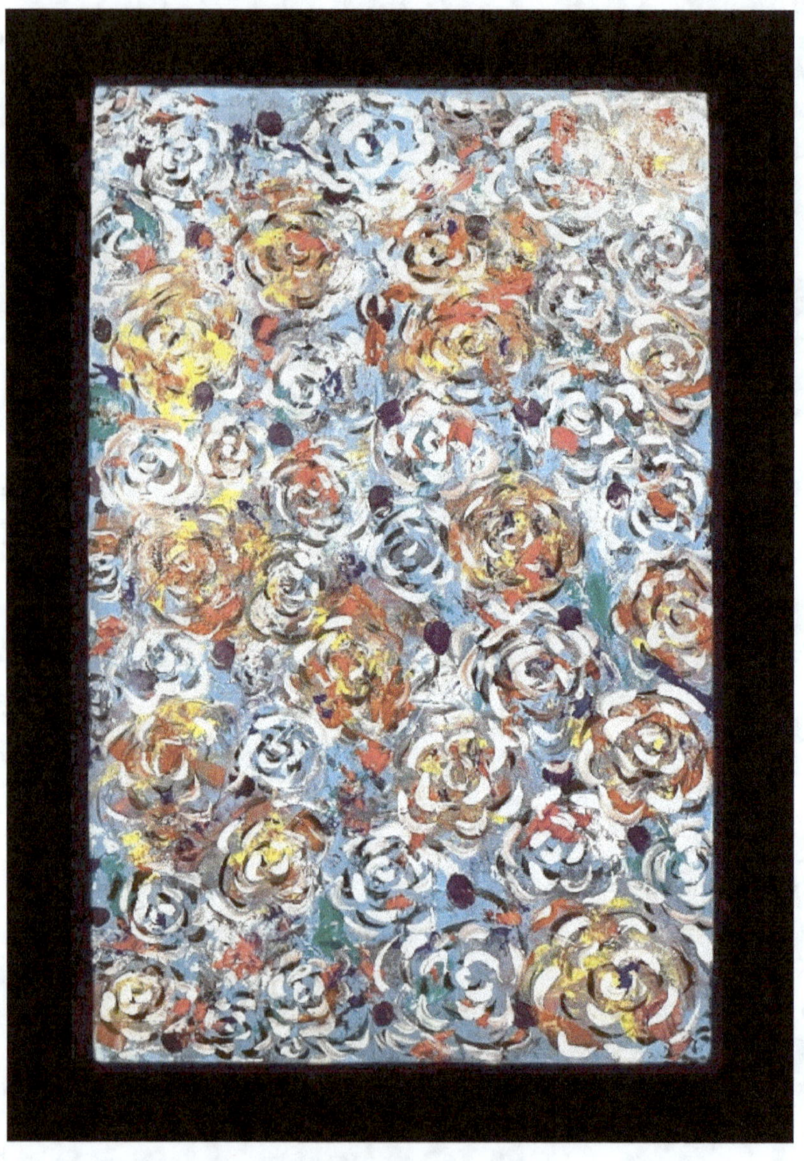

"In a Field of Forever Flowers", Acrylic, 24" x 36", 2023

Salve of Tears

Tonight,
I let my tears
be a balm
for my broken heart.

They wash over me,
cleansing the wounds,
and they beg me,
not to give up.

* * *

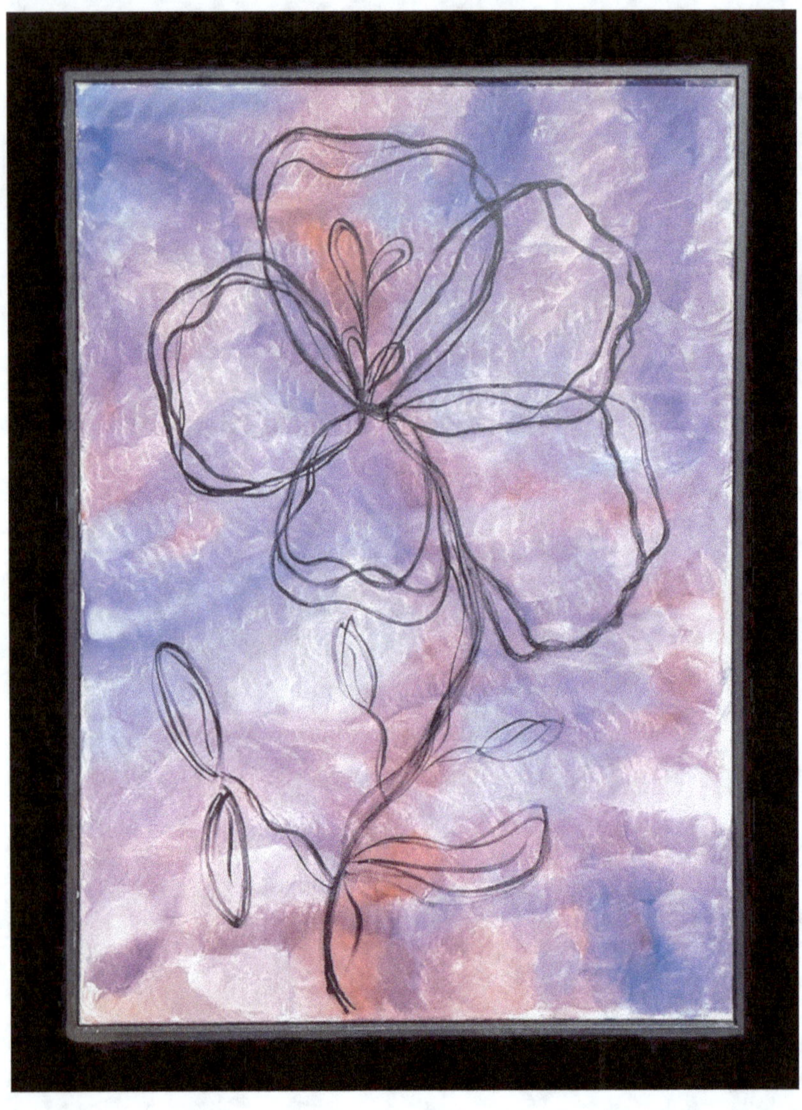

*"**Sunset Thunder**", Oils, 30" x 40", Started 2022, Completed 2023*

Not Too Much to Ask

One day I awoke and said I need more,
Than going alone to the grocery store.
I needed fulfillment, I needed hope,
Because honestly I was at the end of my rope.

I gathered my courage,
To start something new,
It was finally time,
To gain an alternative view.

I pressed forward,
To find more of myself,
I finally took myself,
Off of the damn shelf.

I will no longer settle
For mediocre anymore,
Because there's more to life,
Than cleaning the toys off the floor.

I vow to myself,

To no longer be a shadow,
It's time to embrace me,
It's my time to glow.

***

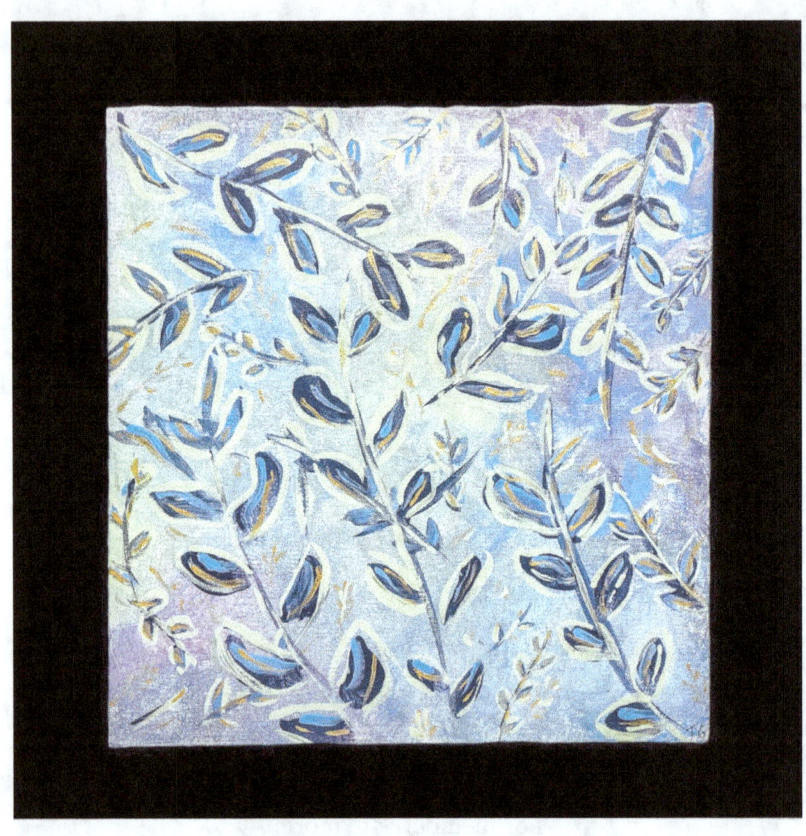

*"**Look up**", Acrylic, 8" x 8", 2023*

Release

It's okay.
You don't have
to carry
that weight
on your shoulders
anymore.

It was never yours
to hold anyway.

Allow it
from your fingers
to fall away.

Let it wash
into the sea
with ease.

There are things
made for you
waiting just beyond
the edge

of the sky.

Release it.
It's time.

* * *

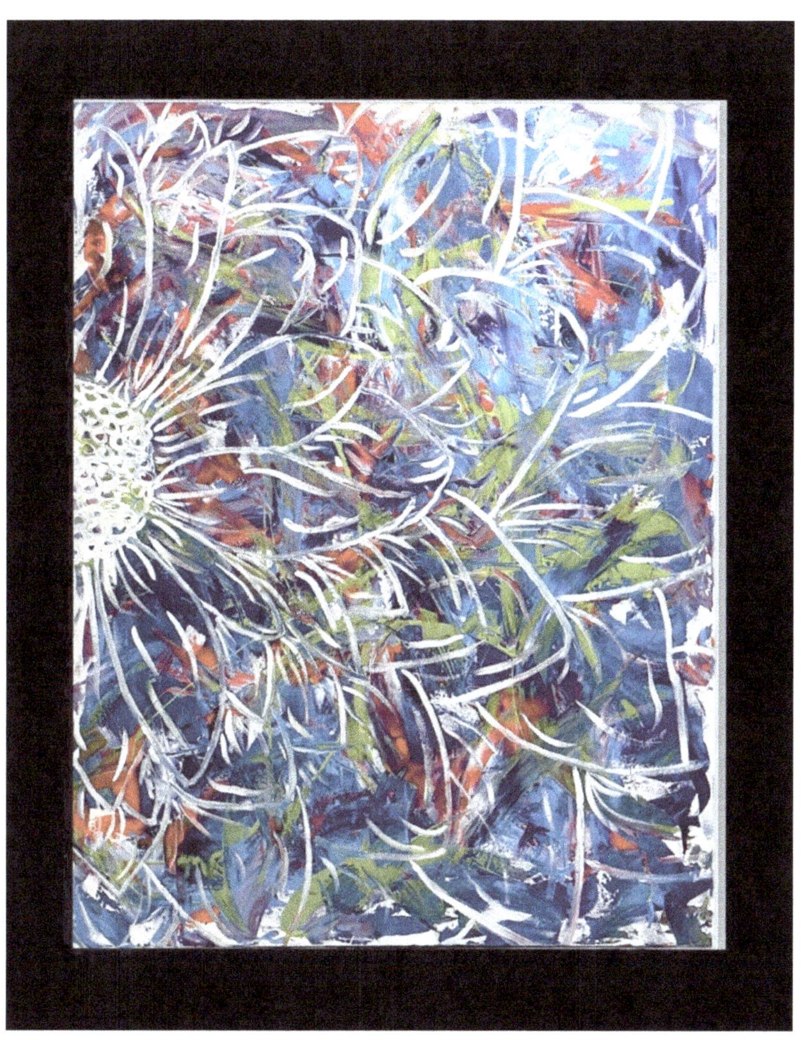

"Oh, She's Wild!", Acrylic, 48" x 60", 2023

Sewing Kit

And for a moment in time,
she felt safe and held,
and she let it mend
a few pieces of her broken heart.

She stitched together
the scraps of her life
that lay tattered and torn
and it began to form a beautiful quilt.

A new colorful vision,
of protection and warmth
lay in her hands.
She had sewn herself once more.

* * *

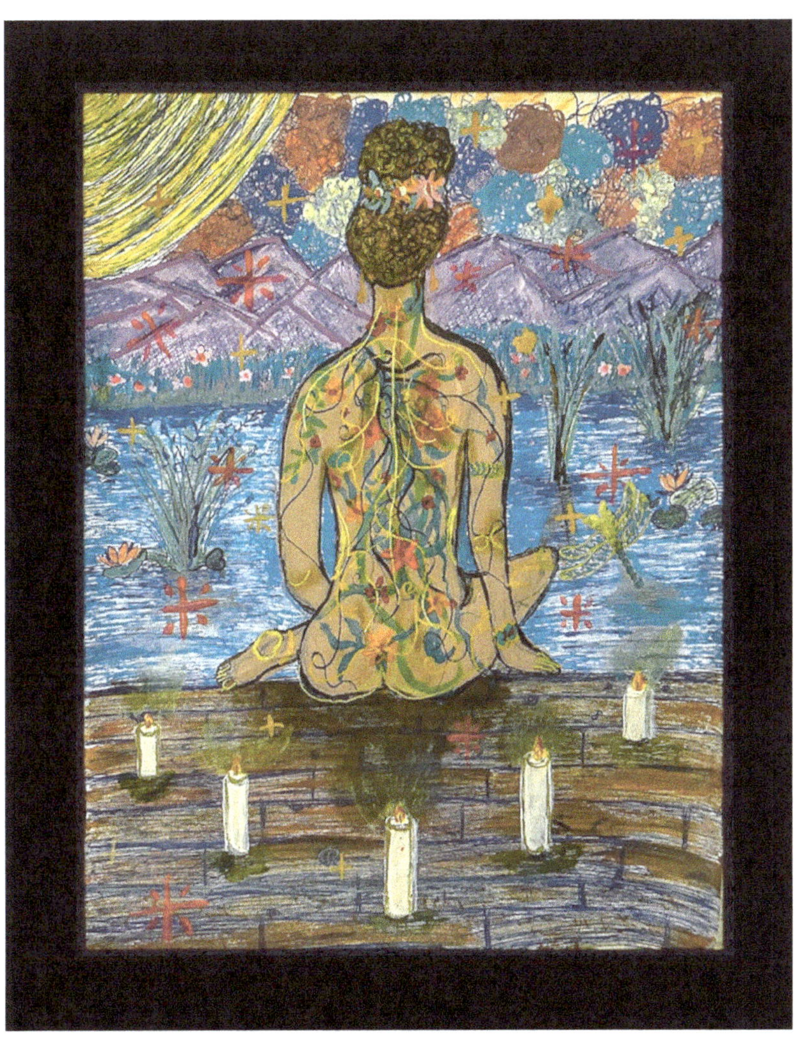

"Finding Myself", Mixed Media, 2024

Love a Little at a Time

I didn't become a mom overnight,
Like they show you in the shows,
It took me well over a year,
Lord only knows.

I had to fight tooth and nail,
For every drop of connection
I had to prioritize self healing,
And deep, difficult reflection.

I was angry it didn't come easy,
Like I always thought it should,
I've learned that even the difficult paths
Can lead to a lot of good.

And though I'm not always,
The mom I wish to be,
My beautiful kiddos
Are the most important people to me.

They are my heart and my soul,
They give my life meaning,

I now look at the incredible humans they are,
And cannot help but beaming.

I wasn't a bad mom,
It was just tough,
But finally I can say,
I am enough!

* * *

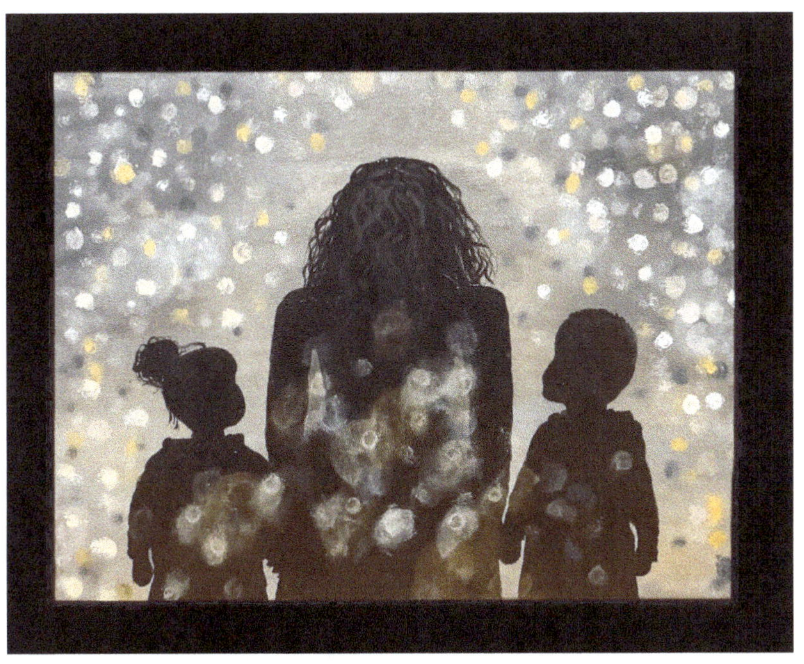

"You and Me Against the World", Acrylic, 18" x 24", 2023

My Garden Finally Grew

For a while my garden shriveled in the heat of motherhood.
The flowers all wilted,
the sun felt too hot,
and vines held me hostage in the weeds.
Yet somehow, I started tasting the rain again.
It moistened my lips, and I drank greedily,
letting the water revitalize my heart.
And the clouds that used to hang distantly in the sky,
moved in a gentle way to offer me shade to rest along the way.

I still often feel like I have a cursed green thumb,
yet my babies are blooming,
despite how much I struggle.
I will not pretend that I didn't think the soil would ever be
rich enough to allow me to grow again,
but I am a column of fire,
flowers,
and exquisite determination to thrive,
and through famine and darkness,
I have survived.

* * *

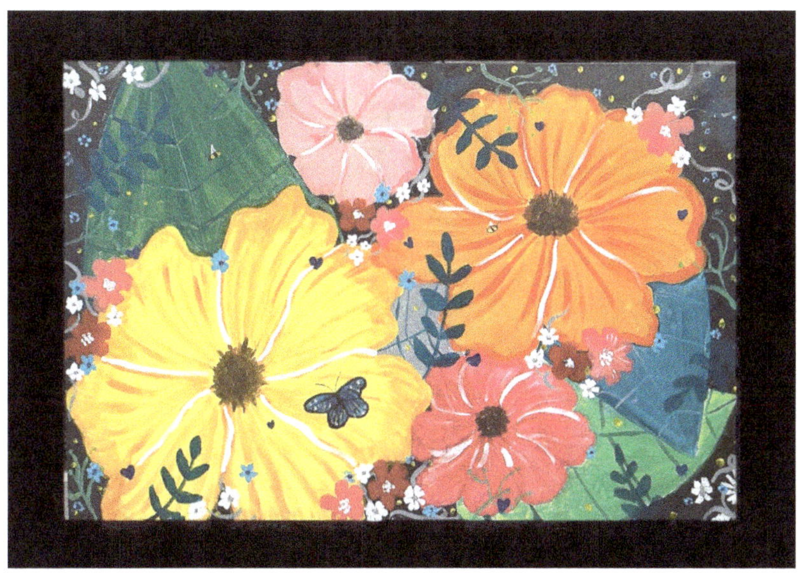

*"**My Happy Garden**", Acrylic, 24" x 36", 2023*

VII

Conclusion

Final Words

It is with my most heartfelt gratitude that I conclude this book. Though I undoubtedly still have healing to do, sharing these thoughts, words and images with you has allowed me to find my voice, my courage, and my determination to find the light. I hope in some small way, maybe it encourages you to do the same.

I would not be here today if it were not for the tremendous support of some amazing people in my life that have walked alongside me, and at times, carried me, while I have weathered this storm. I am so grateful for my dad, my mom, my sister, my family, my beautiful babies, my incredible art and trauma therapists, my team of mental health specialists including my psychiatrist, and all the other women, friends and other good humans who have all made sure that I survived the years immediately following the birth of my children. These years were so tumultuous that I did not want to be here. Thanks to their love, support and unwavering faith in me, I am still here today.

And I am so glad I am.

Regardless of how happy the world tells new moms they should be, it's not always that simple or easy. And if you struggled or you are in the midst of your battle right now, you are not a bad mom for not enjoying every second.

The days may be dark. The nights may feel endless. And you may not feel like yourself for a little while.

But I promise you. You will find the light again.
You are strong. You are worthy of love and support.
And you are a damn good mom!

*A special shoutout to **Mom's Mental Health Initiative** (https://www.mom smentalhealthinitiative.org/) of Wisconsin. They helped me find resources and providers when I was most desperate. I am forever thankful for the ways they helped save my life.*